CHAPTER 1

HUMAN personality is a complex entity, and there have been a multitude of efforts to define and measure it. Most definitions of personality are something like "a collection of emotional, thought and behavioral patterns unique to a person that is consistent over time".

It is common knowledge that personality traits are to a degree heritable. Everybody knows that identical twins are not only "identical" with regard to physical features, but similar in personality as well. And everyone knows instances where a child is a "spitting image" of one of the parents. And by this it is meant that the son or daughter not only looks like, but remarkably behaves like one of the parents.

Scientifically speaking, personality research has not made much progress in the past decades. There are a great many theories of personality, which means that there is no consensus as to which approach is the correct one. Most of the concepts are fuzzy, empirical and not falsifiable.

As things stand at present, the conventional wisdom of the research community is that *many genes* contribute to personality, and the complexity is such that *no gene* contributes more than a few percent of the effect in any aspect of human behavior [Wahlsten, 2012]. As a result, there is currently little effort being made to identify specific genetic personality traits and to incorporate them into a model of personality. The conventional wisdom has firmly established the politically correct illusion that the human personality is so complex that every child is effectively a *tabula rasa* at birth, capable of being molded into any conceivable configuration by parental nurture, education or other aspects of environment.

Unfortunately, the above conventional wisdom is wrong, and it will eventually be shown to be false by geneticists, probably in the not too distant future. In fact, we can easily show that it is false from common experience. We all know of instances where a child has a "personality type" just like one of the parents — who themselves may be very different. It is a very common occurrence. There are striking examples of this in my family and very likely in yours, as well. Now, if *many genes* were involved, a child's inheriting the "entire packet" of personality genes from just one of the parents would be an extremely rare event! After all, the "many" genes would be scattered on that parent's more than twenty pairs of chromosomes, and since a child inherits only one chromosome of each pair, how could "all of the many genes" be transmitted together?

The NPA model of personality traits

The NPA model is the only "trait model of personality" proposed to date that is based on classical genetics [Benis, 1985]. In our experience, the model corresponds closely to reality and explains why so often a child's personality is so similar to that of one of the parents. However, the NPA traits have not yet been researched by geneticists, so results that the model produces must be cautiously termed as theoretical or provisional. But the potential of the NPA model is unique: it is the only theory of personality that proposes to make an assessment of the personality types of children according to the personality types of the parents.

The model was developed on the basis of concepts advanced over seventy years ago by psychiatrist Karen Horney [1950]. According to our model, there are three major, genetically determined, character traits that form the basis of personality. The traits are *sanguinity* (N), *perfectionism* (P) and *aggression* (A). The traits are multifaceted, or in formal terms, each one dependent on a "pleiotropic gene" by which a single gene can cause a complex pattern of characteristics related to behavior.

The letter N is used to denote sanguinity because it is related to the classic concept of "narcissism".

The two traits, A and N, represent the fundamental basis of the human personality structure. Every individual must have a measure of trait A, or trait N, or both.

The genetic basis of an individual's *NPA personality type* is determined by the combination of N, P and A traits that he or she has inherited from the parents. There are about a dozen of the most common NPA personality types. Our premise in this book is that an individual's genetic NPA type can be deduced from analysis of a questionnaire, or "personality test".

The concept that humans have a limited number of discrete character types is not new. Hippocrates in the fourth century B.C. is credited with having developed a scheme of character types based on excesses of body fluids, or "humors". The types emerged under the labels of *Sanguine, Choleric, Phlegmatic* and *Melancholic* (Fig. 1). These types are very close to the personality types generated by our model, especially if one appreciates that the Sanguine and Choleric types represent the fundamental traits of sanguinity and aggression, and that the Phlegmatic and Melancholic types are composites that involve the third trait of the NPA model, perfectionism.

Fig. 1. Character types according to the ancient theory of humors: *Phlegmaticus, Cholericus, Sanguineus* and *Melancholicus. [J.K. Lavater, ca. 1775]* →

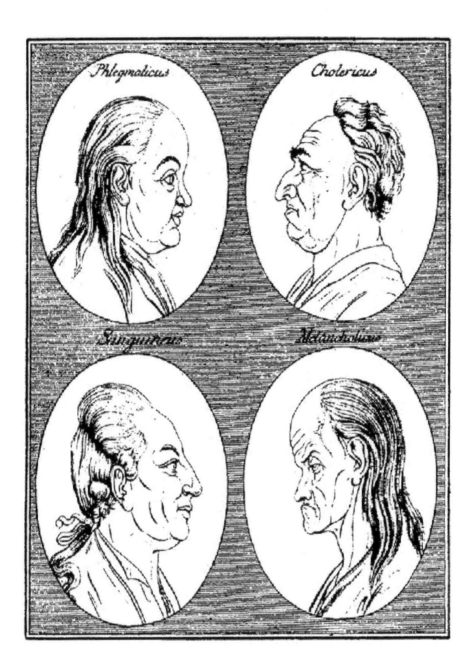

Three traits

Sanguinity (N) is the trait of sociability. Individuals with the trait tend to be prone to flushing, blushing and tearfulness. A hallmark of the trait is the *gingival smile* (Fig. 2) broadly exposing gums and teeth. In the extreme, the N trait appears as a "search for glory", and individuals may display vanity, exhibitionism and show overt narcissistic behavior. Individuals having trait N are called *sanguine types* and sometimes, appropriately, "narcissistic" types.

Fig. 2. The gingival smile. The spontaneous social smile is a hallmark of *sanguinity*, the genetic N trait of the model. →

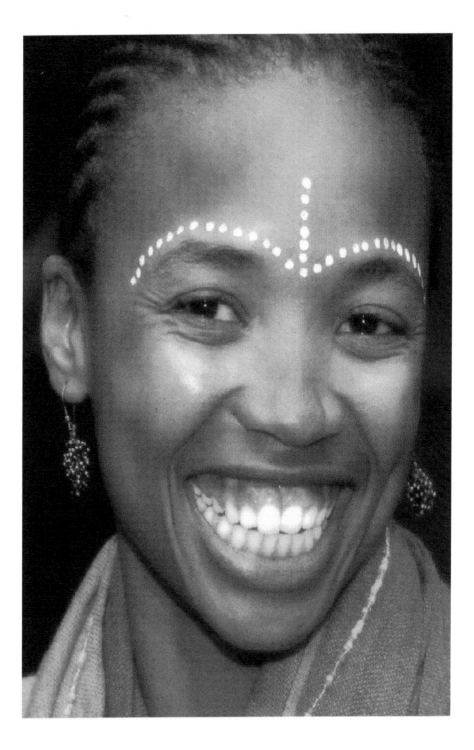

Aggression (A) is the well-known trait of competitiveness, often physical in nature. Individuals having the A trait (but lacking the N trait) tend to be inhibited in sociability and in flushing, blushing, tearfulness and smiling. In the extreme, the trait is a "search for power", and individuals may display physical confrontation, pugnacity and show overtly sadistic behavior. Individuals with the trait of aggression instinctively form "pecking orders". Individuals having trait A, but lacking trait N, are called *non-sanguine* types.

Perfectionism (P) is a trait that may or may not be present in a given individual's NPA type. The trait may be thought of as a modulator of the "unbridled" N and A traits. Individuals having overt expression of the P trait tend to value order, neatness and symmetry, and may be prone to repetitive mannerisms. In the extreme, the trait may be the cause of obsessive-compulsive or autistic-like behavior that may overwhelm other character traits. Individuals lacking trait P are termed *non-perfectionistic*.

Traits A and N are associated with respective rage reactions, namely the classic *aggressive-vindictive rage* (A rage) associated with pallor in individuals of light skin color, and the florid *narcissistic rage* (N rage) associated with sanguinity (Fig. 3). The P trait is not associated with a rage reaction. The traits A and N form the basis of human ambition, namely the desire to achieve power and glory, respectively.

Fig. 3. Faces in rage: the "N rage" in a sanguine type, and "A rage" in a non-sanguine type. →

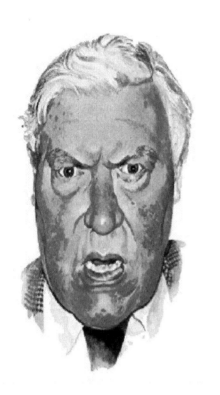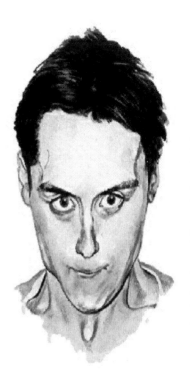

NPA personality types

The model generates a limited number of discrete character types, according to how the three traits are assorted, and whether the traits are present, absent, or incompletely expressed. On the assumption that the three traits are transmitted independently from parents to child, we identify three main categories of personality types: 1) Dominant, 2) Inhibited aggressive, and 3) Borderline types.

In the first category of *Dominant* types the NPA traits are fully expressed. The second category consists of *Inhibited aggressive* types in which the A trait is only partially expressed (Passive aggressive and Resigned types). The third category consists of tenuous *Borderline* types in which neither trait N nor A is fully expressed. Our personality test attempts to identify the more common Dominant and Inhibited aggressive types, as well as less frequently occurring Borderline types.

Dominant types

Here, all three NPA traits are either absent or fully expressed, leading to the following types:

- N   sanguine
- A   non-sanguine aggressive
- NA   sanguine aggressive
- NP   sanguine perfectionistic
- PA   non-sanguine perfectionistic aggressive
- NPA   sanguine perfectionistic aggressive

Types are denoted *sanguine* or *non-sanguine* depending on the presence or absence of the trait N, respectively. The two Dominant non-sanguine types are A and PA.

Types are denoted *aggressive* or *non-aggressive* depending on the presence or absence of the trait A. The two Dominant non-aggressive types are N and NP.

Thus, there are four sanguine and two non-sanguine Dominant types, as well as four aggressive and two non-aggressive Dominant types.

The NP, PA and NPA types are *perfectionistic* types, meaning that they have the P trait. The N, A and NA types are *non-perfectionistic* types. The latter three types, where neither trait N nor A is tempered by the P trait, are prone to what we term "unbridled narcissism" or "unbridled aggression".

In social interactions, a Dominant character type having the A trait has the potential of adopting a *subdued or subjugated state* A− if the particular individual is dominated by a stronger partner. In this state, the Dominant individual would exhibit behaviorisms similar to a Passive aggressive type (see *Inhibited aggression*, below). Similarly, a Passive aggressive type has the potential of being activated to an *energetic state* A+ resembling dominance. Thus, the model emphasizes the potential lability of the A trait, with Dominant and Passive aggressive types continually altering their behavior in competitive interactions with other individuals and in the context of mating. The model emphasizes that from the point of view of inheritance, we need to focus on an individual's baseline genetic NPA type, not on the individual's environmentally influenced social behavior that may vary from day to day.

The N type and the A type may be regarded to be "pure" types, in the sense that they are the only types having just a single NPA trait that is not influenced by the other two traits. Thus, the traits of sanguinity and aggression can be best appreciated in the N and A Dominant types. In these typically extroverted individuals, we can appreciate the unfettered extremes of human behavior that have their roots in the N and A traits. For the N trait, these extremes lie in vanity, exhibitionism and narcissism, or "narcissistic personality disorder". For the A trait, the extremes lie in coerciveness, brutishness and sadism, or "antisocial personality disorder".

The N and A traits are present together, fully expressed, in the NA Dominant type. The two traits tend not to interfere with each other, or modify each other. Rather, they appear together in an unchanged or synergistic manner, so that the NA type is typically an active, highly extroverted, non-perfectionistic individual where full-blown "unbridled" narcissism and aggression are often both on display.

The "bridling" effect of the presence of the P trait on the N and A traits can be profound. The effect on the N trait is such that instead of an outgoing N individual prone to vanity, the result is a less extroverted NP type prone to perfectionistic, obsessive compulsiveness. The effect of the presence of the P trait on the A trait is such that instead of an outgoing A individual prone to overt brutishness, the result is a less extroverted PA type prone to repressed aggressive behavior.

The individual having all three traits together, fully expressed, is the NPA Dominant type (sometimes denoted as the NPA+ type for clarity). This resultant effect of all three traits being present together may be appreciated by imagining "adding the P trait" to the behavior of the NA type. The effect is a tempering one, but the result is still an extroverted individual who may be prone to excesses characteristic of the both the N and A traits acting in concert. The outward effects of the N and A traits may be so overt that although these individuals may consider themselves to be "perfectionists", this may not be the opinion of others. That is, the N and A traits acting together may mask the presence of the P trait as a modulating trait in the sense of the individual's being a "perfectionistic" personality.

Inhibited aggression: Passive aggressive types

If trait A is partially inhibited *genetically from birth*, we obtain the category of Passive aggressive types. The term "Passive aggressive" here simply means that expression of trait A is partially inhibited, and it does not imply "passive-aggressive behavior" in any pejorative sense. We append one minus sign (–) or two minus signs (=) to the letter A, according to whether trait A is only partially or profoundly inhibited.

The model gives us the following Passive aggressive types:

- NPA– NPA= sanguine perfectionistic
- NA– NA= sanguine non-perfectionistic
- PA– PA= non-sanguine perfectionistic
- A– A= non-sanguine non-perfectionistic

Passive aggressive types may be prone to submissive behavior. We designate the A= types *compliant* types and the A– types *non-compliant* types. In dominant-submissive relationships, non-compliant types can play either the dominant or submissive role, depending on the partner, while compliant types will always seek to play the subservient role.

Inhibited aggression in the Passive aggressive types may be best described as the trait of "deference" or "non-confrontation." Although social relationships can be varied and complex, especially when they become stressful, Passive aggressive types tend to gravitate toward avoidance of conflict and to relative deference in social relations.

We noted in the section above that *Dominant types* having the A trait can be reduced to a temporary subdued A− state of relative submission during social interactions, typically when an individual enters into a relationship with a stronger companion. In contrast, in *Passive aggressive types* the A− or A= state is determined from birth by genes and is a stable, baseline trait of relative submissiveness or docility that can be identified in a child at an early age.

Because of the lability of the A trait, non-compliant Passive aggressive types can mimic the A+ state of Dominant types, albeit usually for short periods of time. In this state, for example, the behavior of NA− and NPA− individuals can superficially resemble that of the NA and NPA Dominant types, respectively.

Behaviorisms associated with Passive aggressive types during routine social interactions are similar to those that occur in Dominant types under conditions of stress. These are in the realm of generally restrained behavior, tentative gestures, nervousness and a voice with speech hesitation or tremor.

As in the case of Dominant types, in Passive aggressive types the presence of the P trait can have a profound influence on the expression of the N trait. In the *non-perfectionistic* NA− and NA= types, the N trait may appear in its "unbridled" form as narcissistic flamboyance in dress, gestures and behavior, in a greater tendency to exhibit the gingival smile, and in a higher degree of extroversion. In the *perfectionistic* NPA− and NPA= types, the expression of the N trait is usually well camouflaged because of the modulating effect of the P trait and an accompanying lower degree of extroversion.

Inhibited aggression: Resigned types

If trait A is inhibited because of *environmental constraints after maturity*, we obtain the category of Detachment, or Resignation. Denoting the state of resignation by –A, we obtain the following Resigned types:

- NP –A   sanguine perfectionistic
- N –A   sanguine non-perfectionistic
- P –A   non-sanguine perfectionistic
- –A   non-sanguine non-perfectionistic

Individuals of the Resigned type are mature individuals who previously interacted socially on the basis of the trait of aggression in the context of relationships of dominance and submission.

We identify two groups of Resigned types, namely:

1. former Dominant types (NA NPA PA A), and
2. former non-compliant Passive aggressive types (NA– NPA– PA– A –).

Whereas inhibited aggression in the Passive aggressive types was described as the trait of "deference" or "non-confrontation", in Resigned types it is more in the realm of "avoidance" or "detachment". Because of environmental factors, or "stress", the individual becomes detached, or abdicates from competitive social interaction in order to seek a more serene, independent life style of splendid isolation.

We noted earlier that Dominant types having the A trait and non-compliant Passive aggressive types can vary their status of aggression between A+ and A– states of relative dominance and submission during social interactions. In contrast, the Resigned types, having chosen a life style of independence, actively avoid such interactions as a way of life.

As in the case of the Dominant and Passive aggressive types, the P trait can have a profound tempering influence on the expression of the N trait. In particular, in the non-perfectionistic N –A type, despite an under-lying life style of detachment, the N trait may appear in its unbridled form as unrestrained "narcissism" in dress, in social and sexual behavior, in a greater tendency to exhibit the gingival smile, and generally in a higher degree of extroversion.

Inhibited sanguinity: Borderline non-aggressive withdrawn types

If trait N is inhibited in an *N or NP type* either before or after maturity, we obtain a category of *Non-aggressive withdrawal*. Analogous to the inhibition of trait A presented above, we denote the state of withdrawal by N–, N= and –N as follows:

- N– N= –N   non-aggressive non-perfectionistic
- N– P N= P –NP   non-aggressive perfectionistic

These types are sanguine types, meaning that they have a measure of the N trait even though it is inhibited. They are also by definition *Borderline types*, as they have neither trait N nor A fully expressed.

Borderline types and mental illness

Borderline types possess only one of the traits, N or A, and even that trait is only partially expressed. These types are denoted "borderline" in the sense that they are close to having neither trait N nor A, which according to the model would not be a viable personality type.

Examples of Borderline types would be the A– or PA– Passive aggressive types, –A or P –A Resigned types, or the Non-aggressive withdrawn types described above.

Complexities: other genes and environment

Biological variability and outliers

Just as all males and all females are not alike, there is considerable variability in the behavioral characteristics of a given genetic NPA type. This is basically because of 1) "genes other than the NPA genes" that influence behavior, and 2) environment.

Thus, the NPA traits are only a basic structural skeleton of the human personality, with many other factors, both genetic and environmental, possibly contributing to biological variability in the various NPA types. Among these are *basic drives* (hunger, thirst, sex, territoriality), *cognition* (thinking, learning, reasoning, intelligence), *temperament* (the natural activity or excitability of an individual), as well as other less clearly defined human traits, like empathy and altruism. *Environmental variables* like nurture, culture, and the individual's real-life situation in society provide a final overlay of complexity.

Relationships of dominance and submission

As we emphasized above, in social interactions a Dominant character type having the A trait has the potential of adopting a *subdued or subjugated state* A− if the particular individual is dominated by a stronger partner. In this state, the Dominant individual would exhibit behaviorisms similar to a Passive aggressive type. Similarly, a Passive aggressive type has the potential of being activated to an *energetic state* A+ resembling dominance. Thus, the model emphasizes the potential lability of the A trait, with Dominant and Passive aggressive types continually altering their behavior in competitive interactions with other individuals and in the context of mating.

The model emphasizes that from the point of view of a diagnostic "personality test", we need to focus on an individual's baseline genetic NPA traits, not on the individual's environmentally influenced social behavior that may vary from day to day.

Temperament as a facet of personality

One of the most important aspects of the genetics of personality in the category of "genes other than the NPA genes" is the notion of temperament. By this, we mean the *general activity* or *reactivity* of an individual, in the sense that it is applied with regard to domesticated animals, such as dogs or horses. Thus, a particular individual, say a Dominant NP type, could be described as having a "high temperament" or a "low temperament".

The concept of temperament has not been adequately investigated, or even appreciated, in the behavioral sciences. In the NPA model we make the assumption that the genes that underlie temperament are separate from the NPA genes, hence that the NPA personality type of an individual can be determined irrespective of his or her innate level of temperament. Our NPA personality test makes an effort to measure a subject's level of temperament from the intensity of his or her response to the test questions.

The "television set" analogy

One can think of an individual's personality in terms of the analogy of viewing a television receiver. If there were only two basic models of television sets, then this would represent the *male-female dichotomy*: Then, the *NPA personality type* would then be the channel selector, *temperament* would be the volume control, and how well the TV picture is actually visualized would depend on the lighting in the room, or *environment*.

While acknowledging the complexity of personality in the broader sense, including the above concept of temperament, the model implies that it is the *male-female dichotomy* and the *NPA personality type* that comprise the highest genetic tiers of the human personality structure. Specifically, we assume that despite the complexities of "biological variability" and "temperament", we can, in principle, identify an individual's unique genetic NPA personality type.

Personality tests

Personality assessors based on questionnaires have long been used by researchers in the behavioral sciences, more or less as a last resort. They are not hard science, being used primarily because of the difficulty in quantifying human behavior objectively by any other means. Because of the well-known deficiencies of questionnaire-based assessors, their results must be considered to be provisional — primarily to generate hypotheses that could be subject to confirmation by more rigorous scientific methodology.

As opposed to other approaches, our proposed *NPA personality test* is unique in that it aims to detect the presence or absence of discrete genetic traits, leading to the identification of discrete genetically based personality types. In the chapter that follows, we begin by considering an "idealized NPA test", where idealized subjects of the various NPA personality types always answer the test questions exactly as we expect that they should.

CHAPTER 2

Idealized NPA Personality Test

In this chapter, we present the basic concepts of our approach to a personality questionnaire that aims to identify a subject's NPA type. Our objective at first may appear to be daunting, as there are more than a dozen different NPA types to consider: *Dominant* types, *Inhibited aggressive* types, as well as other less common *Borderline* types.

As a first step toward our objective, we consider an "idealized test" where our subjects always answer the test questions exactly as we expect they should. This simplification allows us to hone the questions to be used in the finalized test, as well as to develop computational techniques for analysis of the results. Later, we will adapt our findings to "real-world" cases in which we retain the same test questions but adapt more comprehensive statistical methods to take into account the fact that individuals of a given NPA type do not always answer the test questions in the same way.

Framework of the test

The test questions

For practical reasons, in order to have an internet-based questionnaire that could be completed in about twenty minutes, we settled on a test consisting of 50 questions, with each question requiring the selection of a numerical integer from 0 to 4 from a dropdown list (five choices). The test questions are reproduced in *Appendix A*. The test is available online in English and five other languages, with scoring by computer being done with the same algorithm for all language versions.

Categorization of questions

Dominant types

The six Dominant types (N, NP, NA, NPA, PA and A) are each allotted 7 questions, for a total of 42 questions, the remaining 8 questions comprising the Passive aggressive/Borderline category of non-dominance (see "S score" below). For details, see *Appendix A*.

For example, in an idealized test an N type would answer positively with "4" for the 7 questions in the N category and "0" for all the other questions. Similarly, an NP type would answer positively with "4" for the 7 questions in the NP category and "0" for all the other questions. And likewise for the other Dominant types.

Passive Aggressive and Borderline types: non-dominance or submissiveness, S score

The eight remaining questions are allotted to the category identifying non-dominant types and the basis of the *S score*, i.e., identifying Passive aggressive and Borderline types. For example, an idealized NA– Passive aggressive type would answer with "4" for both the 7 questions in the NA category and for the 8 questions in the S-score category, answering "0" for all other questions.

The *S score* identifying non-dominance is defined as the sum of the squares of the 8 responses in this category, normalized to a maximum value of 100. Hence, in these idealized tests Passive aggressive and Borderline types have an S score of 100.

Resigned types: detachment, D score

Four questions are allotted to the category identifying Resigned types and the basis of the D score (see *Appendix A*). For example, an N –A Resigned type who was formerly a Dominant type would answer with "4" for both the 7 questions in the NA category and the 4 questions in the Resigned category, answering "0" for all other questions.

The *D score* identifying the Resigned category is defined as the sum of the squares of the 4 responses in this category, normalized to a maximum value of 100. So, in these idealized tests, Resigned types have an D score of 100.

Other scores

Temperament, T score

The *T score* defining "temperament" is taken as the intensity of the subject's response in the Dominant categories of N, A, NA and NPA, defined as the total sum of the squares of the seven responses for all four categories, normalized to a maximum value of 100. We will show below for our idealized cases that elevated scores of $T > 32$ correspond to test results indicating "high-temperament".

Focus, F score

The *F score* defining "focus" is the intensity of the subject's response in the perfectionistic NP and PA categories, defined as the sum of the squares of the seven responses in the two categories divided by the sum of the squares of the total response in all six dominant categories, normalized to a maximum value of 100. So, in the idealized case, a "high-focus" perfectionistic type will have an F score of 100, while a "low-focus" non-perfectionistic type will have an F score of 0.

Extroversion, E score

The *E score* defining "extroversion" is characterized by the subject's positive response in the Dominant NPA category and lack of response in the S category of non-dominance, as defined from the sum of the squares of seven responses in the NPA Dominant category and eight responses in the S score category, normalized to a maximum value of 100. So, for these idealized cases, a "high-extroversion" NPA Dominant type will have an S score of 0 and an E score of 100, while a "low-extroversion" Passive aggressive or Borderline type will have an S score of 100 and an E score of 0.

Analysis of test results for idealized subjects

For the idealized subjects, analysis of the tests is somewhat trivial, since a subject's basic NPA traits are unequivocally revealed by his or her compartmentalized response in only the relevant NPA category. We consider below some issues that will be of use later when we consider the "real world" in which subjects of a given NPA type may not always answer the questions "as expected".

Example 1. Dominant types: test results for the idealized N type

The idealized Dominant N type would answer the questions with a "4" in the seven questions of the N category, and with a "0" to all questions of other Dominant and S categories as follows (reading the 50 answers, left to right):

4 0 0 0 0 0 0 0 0 0 0 0 0 4 0 0 0 0 0 0 4 0 0 0 4

0 0 0 0 0 0 0 0 0 4 0 0 0 4 0 0 0 0 0 0 0 0 0 4 0

For this N type, the normalized *Squares index* for each of the NPA categories is displayed in Fig. 4. The Squares indexes are defined as the sum of the squares of the response values for each of the test question categories, normalized to the maximum value of unity.

Fig. 4. Squares indexes for the different Dominant NPA categories for an idealized N type taking the test. Here, the subject responds positively only to the questions of the Dominant N category, corresponding to a Squares index of 1.00. The value of 0 in the S category identifies the subject to be a Dominant type. →

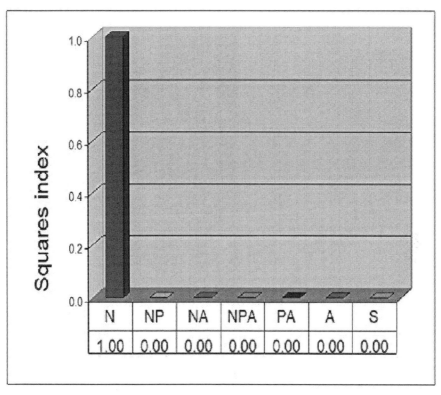

	N	NP	NA	NPA	PA	A	S
	1.00	0.00	0.00	0.00	0.00	0.00	0.00

For the idealized N type, the normalized *Squares index* for the N category is unity, with all other Dominant categories giving values of zero. Thus, for this idealized case, the normalized Squares index of 1.00 is also interpreted to be the *probability* that the test result is consistent with the Dominant N type.

The *Test scores* for the idealized N type are computed to be:

- Non-dominance, $S = 0$
- Detachment, $D = 0$
- Temperament, $T = 25$
- Focus: $F = 0$

Extroversion: $E = 50$

Example 2. Test results for the idealized NP −A Resigned type

As another example, we consider the case of an idealized Resigned type who was a former Passive aggressive NPA− type. This type would answer with a "4" (i.e., *Squares indexes* of unity) for 1) the seven questions of the NP Dominant category, 2) the eight questions of the S category, and 3) the four questions of the Resignation D category. All other questions would get an answer of "0", as follows:

0 0 0 0 4 0 4 0 0 4 4 0 4 0 0 0 0 0 4 4 0 0 4 0 0
0 0 4 4 0 4 4 4 0 0 0 4 0 0 0 4 0 0 4 0 0 4 0 4 0 0 0 0

The *Test scores* for this idealized NP −A Resigned type are:

- Non-dominance, S = 100
- Detachment, D = 100
- Temperament, T = 7
- Focus: F = 82
- Extroversion: E = 0

The S score of 100 identifies the subject as being a non-Dominant type.

Scores for idealized types: Summary

In like manner we can compute the test scores for the other idealized types. These S, D, T, F and E scores are summarized in Table 1 below.

Note to Table 1: scores S, D, T, F and E are normalized arithmetic combinations of the squares of the test answers, while scores A and N are computed from correlation coefficients between the test answers and the answers of the reference Dominant A and N and types, respectively. →

TABLE 1

Test Scores for Idealized NPA types

	S	D	T	F	E	A	N
Dominant							
N	0	0	25	0	50	42	100
NP	0	25	0	100	50	42	42
NA	0	0	25	0	50	42	42
NPA	0	0	25	0	100	42	42
PA	0	0	0	100	50	42	42
A	0	50	25	0	50	100	42
Passive Aggressive							
NA- NA=	100	25	25	0	0	37	37
NPA- NPA=	100	50	0	100	0	37	37
PA- PA=	100	25	0	100	0	37	37
A- A=	100	75	25	0	0	81	37

Resigned, former dominant

N–A	13	100	32	14	44	53	39
NP–A	13	100	32	14	94	53	39
P–A	13	100	7	83	44	53	39
–A	13	100	25	17	44	93	41

Resigned, former passive aggressive

N–A	100	100	32	14	0	47	35
NP–A	100	100	7	82	0	48	36
P–A	100	100	7	83	0	47	35
–A	100	100	25	17	0	79	36

Borderline, non-aggressive, withdrawn

N– N= –N	100	100	32	14	0	47	77
N–P N=P –NP	100	100	7	82	0	48	36

It can be seen from the table that:

- The S and D scores identify whether the test is consistent with a Dominant type or with a non-dominant Passive aggressive, Resigned or Borderline type.
- An elevated focus F score of > 80 indicates the presence of the P trait.
- A low E score of < 50 is consistent with the result of Inhibited aggressive or Borderline type.
- The highest T score for any category is 32. Hence, we consider values of T > 32 to correspond to tests results indicating "high temperament".

Statistical probability: correlation coefficients

In our discussion above, idealized NPA types were identified by their unequivocal responses to the questions in their appropriate NPA categories. In particular, a normalized Squares index of 1.00 indicated that the test was consistent with that particular NPA type with a probability of 1.

Looking forward to the next chapters, where we consider more complicated "real-world" test responses, we introduce a more flexible approach to probability by use of the concept of the *correlation coefficient* (denoted by r), which is a statistical measure of concordance between two fields of numbers, conveniently having a value between +1 and −1. We assume that the 50-point correlation coefficient between a subject's test answers and the answers of a reference test for a particular NPA category is a measure of the *probability* that the test is consistent with that particular category. Specifically, we assume that probability to be r^2 ("r-squared"), which in statistics is known as the *coefficient of determination*.

Example 3. r and r^2 values for the idealized N type

Continuing as in Example 1 above, the test taker once again is an idealized N type who answers the questions with a "4" to the seven questions of the N category, and with a "0" to all other questions.

For this N type, the values of r and r^2 for each of the NPA categories are shown below in Fig. 5 below. These values are represent the 50-point correlation coefficients between the answers of the N type and the answers of each of the 20 idealized NPA categories listed in Table 1.

Fig. 5. Values of r and r^2 for the 20 different NPA categories for an idealized "N type" taking the test. The NPA categories on the x-axis (*left to right*) are divided into the five groups shown in Table 1, as follows: 1) six categories of Dominant types, 2) four categories of Passive aggressive types, 3) four categories of Resigned/former Dominant types, 4) four categories of Resigned/former Passive aggressive types, and 5) two categories of Non-aggressive Borderline types. Positive values of r occur here only for the Dominant N and Borderline N categories. The r^2 values for negative values of r are taken to be 0, corresponding to the nil probability of a positive association in those categories. →

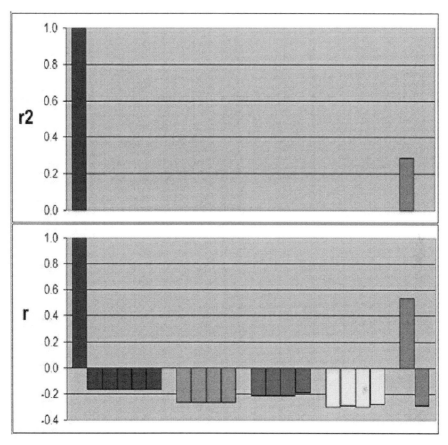

We note the following:

- The values of r and r^2 for the category of "Dominant N type" are 1.00, indicating a perfect correlation of the answers of the idealized N type with the expected answers.
- The values of r for the other five categories of Dominant type (NP, NA, NPA, PA and A) are negative (– 0.16), indicating very poor agreement of the answers with any of the other idealized Dominant types.
- The values of r for the next three groups of four categories (Passive aggressive, Resigned/former Dominant, Resigned/ former Passive aggressive) are likewise negative, indicating again very poor agreement of the answers of the N type with any of these idealized types.

- The value of r for the last group of two categories (Non-aggressive Borderline types) is positive only for the non-perfectionistic sanguine types such as N−. The values of r and r^2 here are 0.54 and 0.29 respectively. Thus, the test results are interpreted to be compatible only with the Dominant N type or with the Borderline N type, in a probability ratio of their respective r^2 values, or 1 : 0.29.

Example 4. r and r^2 values for the idealized NP type

As another example, the test taker here is an idealized NP type who answers the questions with a "4" in the seven questions of the NP category, and with a "0" to all other questions.

For this NP type, the values of r and r^2 for each of the NPA categories are shown in Fig. 6, below. These values represent the 50-point correlation coefficients between the answers of the idealized NP type and the answers of each of the 20 idealized NPA categories listed in Table 1.

Fig. 6. Values of r and r^2 for the 20 different NPA categories for an idealized NP type taking the test. The five groups of NPA categories on the x-axis are the same as those depicted in Fig. 5. Here, positive values of r occur (from left to right) only for the categories of 1) Dominant NP, 2) Passive aggressive NPA−/NPA=, 3) Resigned/former Passive aggressive NP −A, and 4) Borderline NP. →

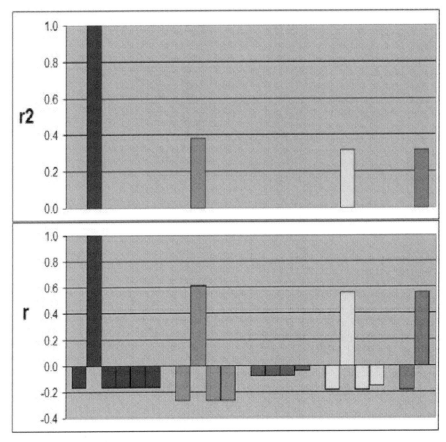

We note the following:

- The values of r and r^2 for the category of "Dominant NP type" are 1.00, indicating a perfect correlation of the answers of the idealized NP type with the expected answers.

- The values of r for the other five categories of Dominant type (N NA NPA PA A) are negative (− 0.16), indicating very poor agreement of the answers with any of the other idealized Dominant types.

- The values of r in the other four groups of non-dominant types are positive only for the categories of Passive aggressive NPA−/NPA=, Resigned/former Passive aggressive NP−A, and Borderline NP, these values being 0.62, 0.62 and 0.56, respectively. The corresponding r^2 values are: 0.38, 0.32 and 0.32.

- Thus, results are interpreted to indicate that the test answers are compatible only with the types Dominant NP, Passive aggressive NPA−/NPA=, Resigned NP−A and Borderline NP in probability ratios of their respective r^2 values, or 1 : 0.38 : 0.32 : 0.32.

Aggression and Sanguinity scores from correlation coefficients

Use of the correlation coefficient, r, allows us to define A and N scores, which give a measure of how closely a subject's test response matches the answers of the reference tests of the "unbridled" A and N Dominant types.

For a given test, we define scores for *Aggression* and *Sanguinity* as computed from 50-point correlations of the test answers with the reference categories of the Dominant A type for the A score, and the Dominant N type for the N score. The A and N reference categories represent "unbridled" aggression or "unbridled" sanguinity, where the A and N traits are not modulated by the P trait. Thus, high values of the A or N score could be indicative antisocial aggression or narcissism.

Aggression, A score

The *A score* of a test is taken to be proportional to the r value corresponding to the correlation of the test answers with the reference test answers of the idealized A type. The score is normalized to a scale of 0 to 100, corresponding to r values of -1 and $+1$, respectively. Values of the A score for the idealized NPA types are given in Table 1. It can be seen that the A score for the idealized NPA types is below 55 except for the Dominant, Inhibited aggressive and Borderline A types.

Sanguinity or Narcissism, N score

The *N score* of a test is taken to be proportional to the r value corresponding to the correlation of the test answers with the reference test answers of the idealized N type. The score is normalized to a scale of 0 to 100, corresponding to r values of -1 and $+1$, respectively. Values of the N score for the idealized NPA types are given in Table 1. It can be seen that the N score for the idealized NPA types is below 45 except for the Dominant and Borderline N types.

Summary of idealized test

- The idealized NPA personality test consists of 50 questions, each question requiring a numerical answer from 0 to 4 (five choices).

- The 50 questions are divided into six categories of Dominant types (N NP NA NPA PA A), and a seventh group (S) defining non-dominance or Submissiveness.

- Four categories of Passive aggressive types are characterized with the use of the S *score*.

- In addition, eight categories of Resigned types and two categories of Non-aggressive Borderline types are defined with the use of the S score and a Detachment D *score*.

- In an idealized test, a subject of a given NPA type chooses the maximum response of "4" for the questions in the appropriate test question categories and the null response of "0" for all other questions.

- Besides the S and D scores, three other test scores are defined for Temperament (T *score*), Focus (F *score*) and Extroversion (E *score*). The above five scores are computed as arithmetic combinations of the squares of the test answers. All scores are scaled from 0 to 100.

- A *Squares index* for each of the test question categories is defined as the sum of squares of the test answers, normalized to a maximum value of 1. Idealized NPA types obtain Squares indexes of 1 in the appropriate categories, this being interpreted as the ideal probability of 1 that the test answers are consistent with that NPA type.

- A more practical parameter is introduced for the comparison of a subject's test answers and those of a reference test, namely the *correlation coefficient*, r. We assume that the probability of concordance between the subject's test and a reference test is the r^2 value, or *coefficient of determination*.

- The correlation coefficient allows us to introduce two additional scores. These are the Aggression A *score* and the

Sanguinity/Narcissism *N score*. Each is defined with the use of the idealized answers of the A and N Dominant types, respectively, and their coefficients of correlation with the subject's test answers. Both scores are scaled from 0 to 100.

- The analysis in the present chapter is confined to idealized cases in which subjects of particular NPA type categories uniformly give test answers exactly matching their expected reference values. In the next chapter we consider the more general "real-world" cases where this rarely occurs.

CHAPTER 3

Real-world NPA Personality Test

In this chapter, we refine our approach to the final version of a test that aims to diagnose a subject's NPA type. In the previous chapter, we considered the idealized situation in where a test taker answered positively only to questions of a single NPA category. Here, we consider the real-world situation where a test taker of a particular NPA type may answer positively in other test question categories, as well.

Framework of the test

The test questions

The test uses the same 50 questions that we presented in the idealized version, again with each question requiring the selection of a numerical integer from 0 to 4 (five choices). The test questions are reproduced in *Appendix A*.

Categorization of questions and analysis

In the previous chapter, we presented a method of analysis for *idealized tests* in which we proposed:

- Categorization of idealized NPA types according to our personality model. Twenty NPA categories were proposed, including six Dominant types, and fourteen more Inhibited aggressive and Borderline types
- Use of a set of idealized test answers for each idealized NPA category, to be used as "reference tests"
- Selection of the most probable diagnosis for a test according to how well the subject's test answers correlate with the set of reference tests (r and r^2 values).

Our analysis of real-world tests is the same as that presented for the idealized types with the following modifications:

- Instead of the 20 idealized reference tests, we use a total of 19 tests, each of which is a *composite of actual tests* that we have received for the various presumed NPA categories.
- We employ a computerized algorithm that uses not only the correlation coefficient (r), but also other measures of statistical concordance to select the best match between the subject's test answers and the reference tests.
- We introduce two additional statistical scores based on correlation coefficients: the *R score* and the *C score*.

The Standard Reference tests

The 19 Standatrd tests are listed below. Each test is a composite of from 4 to 10 actual tests in which each of the 50 answers is an average.

N group

1. Dominant N type with low S score
2. N or NA− type with low-moderate S score
3. N type with high-moderate S score, or Borderline N type

NP group

1. Dominant NP type with low S score
2. Passive aggressive type, NPA− /= with high S score
3. Passive aggressive type, NPA− /= with high S score & PA index

NA group

1. Dominant NA type with low S score
2. Dominant NA type with higher S score
3. NA or NA− /= type with very high S score
4. NA or NA− /= type with very high S score & high PA index
5. NA−/NA= or N with high S score, low NP index
6. NA−/NA= or N with moderate S score & high NP index

NPA group

1. Dominant NPA type with low S score
2. Dominant NPA type with higher F score
3. Dominant NPA type with higher F score

PA group

1. Dominant PA type with low S score
2. Dominant PA type with higher S score

A group

1. Dominant A type with low S score
2. Dominant A type with lower T, higher F score

Characteristics of the Standard tests

Squares indexes

The Standard tests are displayed graphically in Fig. 7, below. Each panel shows the Squares indexes for the seven NPA categories into which the test questions were partitioned (see *Appendix A*).

Fig. 7. The 19 Standard Reference tests, grouped according to their diagnostic NPA types. The graphs show the *normalized Squares indexes* according to the seven categories into which the test questions were divided (N NP NA NPA PA A & S). →

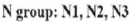

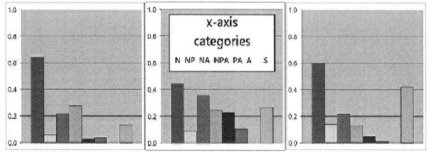

NP group: NP1, NP2, NP3

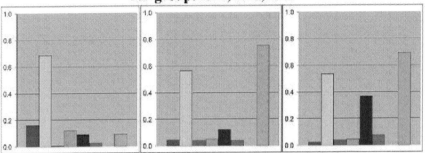

NA group: NA1, NA2, NA3, NA4, NA5, NA6

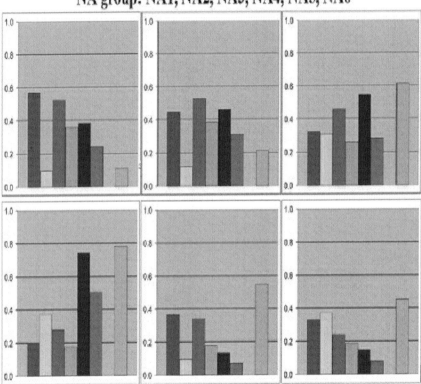

NPA group: NPA1, NPA2, NPA3

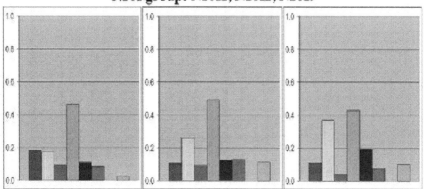

PA group: PA1, PA2

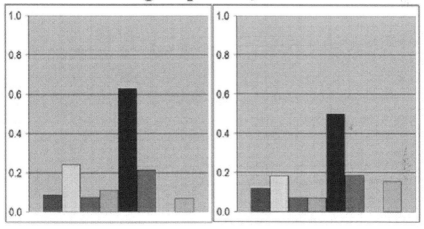

A group: A1, A2

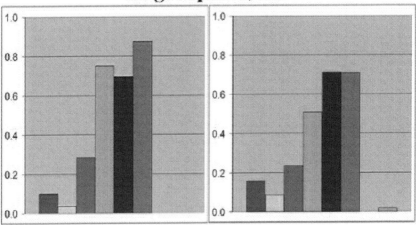

One can see from Fig. 7 that the Standard tests differ from the Idealized reference tests used in Chap. 2. in three ways:

- In none of the Standard tests does a Squares index approach the idealized value of unity.
- A Standard test in a given NPA group may have non-zero Squares indexes in several other NPA categories.
- For a Standard test in a given NPA group, the maximum value of the Squares index need not correspond to the same NPA category as that of the group.

One can see for the NA group, for example, that the maximum value of the Squares index for Standard test NA4 is not of the NA category, but of the PA category.

Test scores

Test scores for the Standard tests are summarized in Table 2, below. One can see that the S scores for the tests range from 0 to 78.

The tests corresponding to the *Dominant* NPA types (low S scores, ranging from 0 to 21) are: N1, NP1, NA1/NA2, NPA1/NPA2/NPA3, PA1/PA2 and A1/A2.

Table 2 below summarizes the nine different *Test scores* for each

Standard test (See *Appendix A*). →

TABLE 2. Test scores for the Standard Reference Tests

	test	S	D	T	F	E	A	N	R	C
1	N1	13	3	30	10	66	32	100	100	87
2	N2	27	23	29	28	56	40	93	100	89
3	N3	42	11	24	23	39	16	90	100	93
4	NP1	9	20	8	77	55	21	52	100	90
5	NP2	75	37	4	85	16	11	42	100	91
6	NP3	69	39	5	87	19	22	28	100	87
7	NA1	11	21	42	25	73	75	77	100	85
8	NA2	21	29	45	27	70	75	74	100	80
9	NA3	62	37	33	42	40	47	42	100	80
10	NA4	78	51	29	51	25	49	11	100	61
11	NA5	55	18	24	26	37	24	82	100	95
12	NA6	45	30	21	46	42	14	74	100	95
13	NPA1	3	6	21	34	86	66	70	100	77
14	NPA2	11	17	20	40	83	49	60	100	81
15	NPA3	10	22	16	54	79	42	58	100	87
16	PA1	7	46	12	70	55	83	13	100	86
17	PA2	15	42	11	68	48	76	12	100	63
18	A1	0	45	50	28	100	100	32	100	95
19	A2	2	44	40	36	90	100	28	100	94

The statistical functions

Our test algorithm is a logical scheme based on statistical methods that uses various criteria to decide the best concordance between the subject's test answers and the answers corresponding to the Standard tests.

The algorithm uses the following statistical functions:

- the Squares indexes
- the r and r^2 functions
- the J-function
- the Z-function
- the rho and rho-squared functions

- the kappa and kappa-squared functions.

The Squares indexes and the r and r^2 functions

The Squares indexes were presented in Chap. 2. and are the basis of the values displayed in the panels of Fig. 7, above. The r and r^2 functions (based on the correlation coefficient and the coefficient of determination) were also introduced in Chap. 2.

The J-function

The J-function is defined as the reciprocal of the *sum of the squares of the differences* between the test answers and the answers of each of the 19 Standard tests. As with the r^2 values, the relative probability of concordance between the subject's test and a Standard test is presumed to be proportional to the magnitude of the J-function.

Analysis of the sum of the squares of the differences between two sets of numbers, as in the J-function, is similar to the basis of the classical "chi-square test" used in statistics.

The Z-function

The Z-function is defined as the reciprocal of the *variance* of the differences between the subject's answers and the answers of each of the 19 Standard tests. The relative probability of concordance between the subject's test and a Standard test is presumed to be proportional to the magnitude of the Z-function.

In statistics, the square root of the variance is the well-known *standard deviation*. The J, Z and r functions are closely related. In fact, values of Z and r can be calculated directly from a J value, provided that one knows for a set of paired values 1) the mean difference between the two fields, and 2) the variance of each field. (It is not necessary to know the individual values of each field.) Nevertheless, values of J, Z and r for sets of paired values are generally not proportional, and the three functions will give different relative results.

The rho and rho-squared functions

Values of the *rho-function* are 19-point correlation coefficients between the set of r values for the subject and for each of the Standard tests. Thus, the rho-function compares the "fingerprints" of r values between the subject and each of the nineteen Standard tests. As with squared values of the r-function, values of *rho-squared* are assumed to be proportional to the probability of concordance between a subject's test and a Standard test.

The kappa and kappa-squared functions

Values of the *kappa-function* are 19-point correlation coefficients between the set of J values for the subject and for each of the Standard tests. Thus, the kappa-function compares the "fingerprints" of J values between the subject and each of the nineteen Standard tests. As with squared values of the r and rho functions, values of *kappa-squared* are assumed to be proportional to the probability of concordance between a subject's test and a Standard test.

Statistical agreement: the R and C scores

In the previous chapter, use of the correlation coefficient, r, allowed us to define A and N scores, which give a measure of how closely a subject's test response matches the answers of the reference tests of the Dominant A and N types. Here we define two other scores, the R score and the C score, which describe aspects of the statistical consistency of a subject's response to the questions (see also *Appendix A*).

R score

The R score of a test, denotes "consistency of response to questions," or "coherence". It is computed from the maximum value plus the standard deviation of the 19 values of the r-function. Thus, if a subject gives test answers (0 to 4) in a completely random fashion, the 19 values of the correlation coefficient r will cluster around 0 with a very small standard deviation. The possible range of values of R is scaled from 0 to 100. A value of R of less than 50 is unusual and can have many possible explanations. Whatever the reason for a low score, it indicates that the subject responded "exceptionally", in the sense of his or her test result not having a high correlation with any of the 19 Standard reference tests.

C score

The C score of a test, denotes "statistical consistency", as determined by the correlation coefficient between the 19 pairs of values of the rho and kappa functions. Since the rho and kappa functions depend on the r and J functions, respectively, the C score is taken as a measure of how well the four statistical computations agree. The C score of 0 is scaled from 0 to 100, with the zero value corresponding to a zero or negative correlation coefficient.

The test algorithm

Our test algorithm is uses Boolean logic and the statistical functions described above to decide the best concordance between the subject's test answers and the answers corresponding to the Standard tests.

The algorithm has the following features:

- It attempts to identify a most likely NPA category consistent with the Standard tests, assigning it a *relative probability* of 1.
- It uses weighted averages values of the Squares index, and the r^2, J, Z, rho-squared and kappa-squared functions.
- It uses acceptability criteria for each NPA type, including ones based on the test Scores (S, D, T, etc.).
- It uses criteria to identify the lesser likely NPA categories, assigning them a lower relative probability of agreement.

Example 5. Comparison of the r^2, J, Z, rho-squared and kappa-squared functions

As an example to illustrate our use of the various statistical functions, we present a real-world test from our archives.

The subject was a female, age 31 to 40, who did not specify any disease or other condition and did not otherwise comment. Her submitted test answers were:

3 2 4 2 1 2 0 0 0 2 0 4 3 4 2 4 4 0 4 0 4 0 1 0 1
0 2 0 0 3 0 0 1 0 3 1 0 1 1 2 0 0 1 0 3 2 1 3 4 0

The normalized *Squares index* for each of the test question categories is displayed in Fig. 8, below. The Squares indexes are calculated, as usual, as the sum of the squares of the response values for each of the NPA question categories, normalized to the maximum value of unity. Also shown below are the test scores for this test.

Fig. 8. Example 4: Values of the Squares index for the seven categories into which the questions are partitioned. →

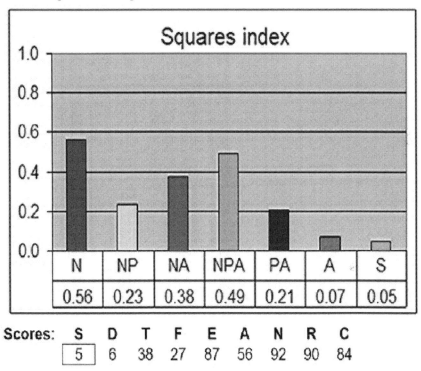

Scores:
S	D	T	F	E	A	N	R	C
5	6	38	27	87	56	92	90	84

One can see that with a low S score of 5 that the subject is a diagnosed to be a Dominant type. The highest Squares index is in the N category, but the subject also scored significantly in the other categories, as well.

We now make us of our Standard reference tests. In Fig. 9 we display the values of the r^2, J, Z, rho-squared and kappa-squared functions for each of the 19 Standard tests. The x-axis categories are those of the 19 tests, in the same 6 groups (N, NP, NA, NPA, PA and A) and in the same order as detailed previously in Fig. 7 and Table 2. The graphs in Fig. 9 show clearly that the five statistical functions, although closely related, do not give proportional numerical results.

Fig. 9. *From top to bottom:* the r^2, J-function, Z-function, rho-squared and kappa-squared values for each category of the 19 Standard tests. For purposes of comparison, the maximum value in each panel (the N1 Standard test category) has been normalized to a value of unity. →

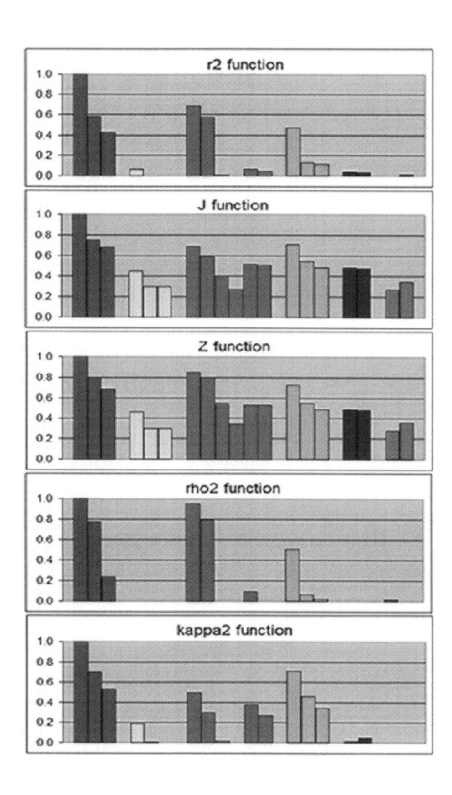

Display of results in this book

As it would be onerous to try to include all the details of the statistical functions for every test that we present, in the remainder of this book we confine ourselves to display of the results in abridged form as shown in Fig. 10 below. The data in this figure are a condensation of the results just presented in Example 5, above.

Fig. 10. Display of test results in abridged form. →

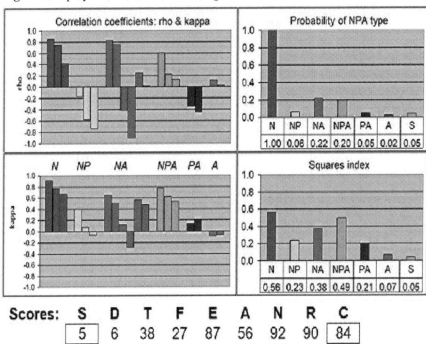

The abridged results include the following:

- *Upper right panel:* the probability of concordance with one of the Standard test categories, as determined by the test algorithm. The highest probability is given the value of unity.
- *Lower right panel:* the Squares indexes, according to the seven groups into which the 50 test questions are partitioned.
- *Panels at left:* the correlation coefficients rho and kappa.
- *Below:* the nine Test scores, S D T F E A N R C

As to the results for Example 5 summarized in Fig. 10 above, we see that the algorithm chose "Dominant N type" as the diagnosis having the highest probability, despite the moderate rho/kappa correlation with the Standard tests in the NA and NPA categories. The relatively high C score of 84 indicates that the statistical agreement between the rho and kappa functions was satisfactory in this case.

CHAPTER 4

Dominant types
N NP NA NPA PA A

Case 1 "Idealized" N type

4 0 0 0 0 0 0 0 0 0 0 0 0 4 0 0 0 0 0 0 4 0 0 0 4

0 0 0 0 0 0 0 0 0 0 4 0 0 0 4 0 0 0 0 0 0 0 0 4 0

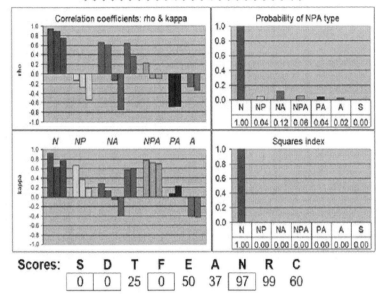

Scores:

S	D	T	F	E	A	N	R	C
0	0	25	0	50	37	97	99	60

The idealized Dominant N type (see Chap. 2) answers the questions with a "4" for the seven questions of the N category, and with a "0" to all other questions in the other Dominant and S categories.

The normalized *Squares index* for each of the NPA categories is displayed above. The Squares indexes are calculated as the sum of the squares of the response values for each of the test question categories, normalized to the maximum value of unity. The graph shows that the normalized Squares index for the N category is 1.00, with all the other categories giving values of zero.

Diagnosis: N type

As expected, the test algorithm had no difficulty making the diagnosis of Dominant N type (graph at upper right). Both the rho and kappa correlation coefficients are highest for the N1 category (first red bar in the graphs at left, with values on the order of 0.94). The S score is 0, indicating a Dominant type. The detachment D and focus F scores are also 0, indicating 1) no tendency to social detachment, and 2) an NPA type lacking the trait P.

The N score of 97 is close to its maximum value of 100. The C score of 60 indicates a fair agreement between the sets of the rho and kappa correlation coefficients.

2 Actual test, very close to the "idealized" N type

4 0 0 0 0 0 0 0 0 0 0 0 0 0 0 4 0 0 0 0 4 0 0 0 0

0 0 0 0 0 0 0 0 0 0 0 0 0 0 4 0 0 0 0 0 0 0 0 4 0

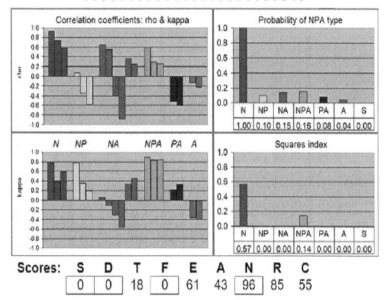

Scores:	S	D	T	F	E	A	N	R	C
	0	0	18	0	61	43	96	85	55

The subject is female, age 21 to 30.

It is an unusual test. The subject answered with a "4" to four of the questions in the N category and to one question in the NPA category, and "0" to all other questions. (Note that for the questions given a "0" value, the subject needed to enter a "0"; the questions were not just ignored.) It is as if the subject had decided, "I will answer with a "4" only to those questions with which I agree 100%, and "0" to all other questions."

The normalized Squares indexes for the NPA categories are displayed above. The graph shows that the Squares index for the N category is 0.57 and 0.14 for the NPA category.

Diagnosis: N type

Again, the test algorithm chose the diagnosis of Dominant N type (graph at upper right). The highest correlation coefficient was for rho in the N1 category (first red bar in the graphs at left, value of 0.93). The S score is 0, indicating a Dominant type. The detachment D and focus F scores are also 0, indicating 1) no tendency to social detachment, and 2) an NPA type lacking the trait P.

The N score of 96 is close to its maximum value of 100. The C score of 55 indicates only fair agreement between the sets of rho and kappa correlation coefficients.

3 N type, opera singer

3 0 1 3 1 2 0 0 1 0 0 0 3 4 1 4 3 0 2 0 3 0 0 3 1
1 1 0 1 1 0 0 2 2 1 3 1 3 1 4 0 0 0 1 4 1 2 0 4 0

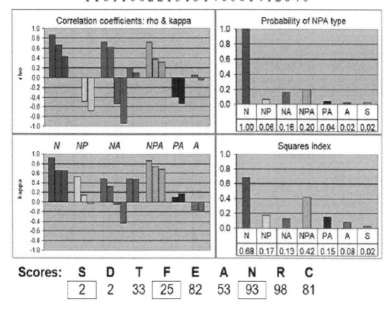

Scores:

S	D	T	F	E	A	N	R	C
2	2	33	25	82	53	93	98	81

The subject is female, age 21 to 30. Migraine headaches. *I don't see why this test wouldn't be accurate. The S-score is dead on. One problem, though: I am an opera singer, so asking about roles made it harder for me to answer some questions. I would have to act a certain way if the part required it, wouldn't I?*

Diagnosis: N type

The test shows Dominant N type with very low S score (2) and high N score (93). The temperament T score is moderate (33), while the extroversion E score is on the high side (82), indicating an outgoing, sociable individual. As would be expected for a non-perfectionistic personality type, the focus F score is low (25).

Dominant N types typically take pride in having a low S score and high E score on the test.

The "N type" would be a common type for an opera singer, as well as for other branches of the performing arts.

4 N type with exceptional intellectual and artistic gifts

3 1 1 2 2 0 1 1 2 0 1 3 2 3 0 1 3 1 2 1 4 0 2 3 3
0 3 0 1 1 3 1 1 1 3 2 2 0 2 4 3 0 0 3 3 2 1 2 2 1

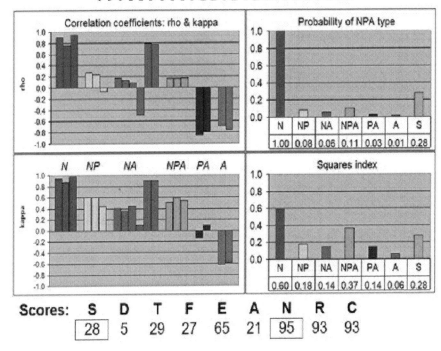

Scores:	S	D	T	F	E	A	N	R	C
	28	5	29	27	65	21	95	93	93

The subject is female, age 41-50. Asthma, *My narcissism lies in my intellectual and artistic gifts... but since other people appreciate these talents, I don't feel like a raving egomaniac for no reason.*

Diagnosis: N type

The test shows Dominant N type with low S score (28) and high N score (95). The temperament T and extroversion E scores are moderate (29, 65), indicating a sociable individual of medium temperament. As would be expected for a non-perfectionistic personality type, the focus F score is low (27).

The subject is a bit defensive regarding the possible vulnerability to "narcissism" in a Dominant N type. We can translate her comment as *"Yes, I know that other people notice that I behave like a narcissistic, raving egomaniac, but deep down they appreciate my extraordinary intellectual and artistic gifts, so I have no reason to try to restrain myself."*

Indeed, a major vulnerability of the N type is to overt narcissism and to displays of vanity. In their comments, N types sometimes wish to convey to us that they are endowed with extraordinary physical attributes, or with exceptional or magical qualities of behavior and insight.

5 NP type with ADD and OCD tendencies

0 1 0 2 3 3 1 0 0 0 1 2 3 0 0 0 0 0 0 0 1 0 2 0 0
2 0 2 3 0 4 0 2 1 2 0 2 0 0 0 1 0 0 1 1 0 0 0 0 0

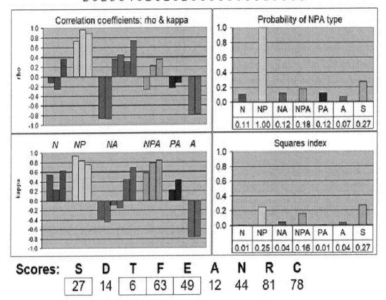

Scores:	S	D	T	F	E	A	N	R	C
	27	14	6	63	49	12	44	81	78

The subject is female, age 31-40. ADD, attention deficit disorder. *I think the test was extremely accurate, as close to 100% as I feel you can get with this type of test. I'm fairly certain that my father is also an NP, while I suspect that my mother was most likely a BPD* [Borderline Personality Disorder]... *I believe 'most' of my OCD tendencies and my normal control tendencies (marriage issues excluded) are coping mechanisms for ADD. Most of these behaviors I developed at a young age to deal with the anxieties of having ADD and sort of behavior modification.*

Diagnosis: NP type

The test shows Dominant NP type with a low S score (27). As would be expected for an NP type with obsessive-compulsive behavior (or OCPD), the focus F score is > 50. The temperament T and extroversion E scores are low (14, 49), suggesting a sociable, but reserved, individual.

The father's also being an NP type would be consistent with the NPA model, by which any NP type must have at least one parent who is either an N or NP type [Benis, 1985]. The subject's detailed comment with correct capitalization and punctuation also speaks for highly expressed P trait typically seen in the NP type. The ADD diagnosis is unusual in the NP type, but it does occur. In our English language series, 3 out of 100 subjects giving the diagnosis of ADD tested as Dominant NP type.

6 NP type, parent of child with autism

0 0 0 0 0 0 2 0 2 0 0 2 4 0 0 2 0 0 0 2 0 0 3 1 0
0 0 4 2 4 0 0 0 0 0 4 0 0 0 0 0 0 0 3 3 2 0 0 0 0

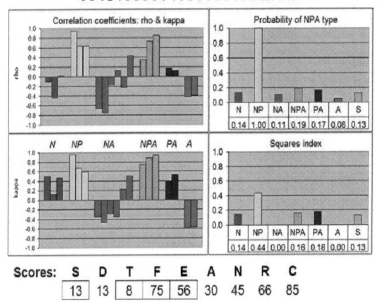

Scores:

S	D	T	F	E	A	N	R	C
13	13	8	75	56	30	45	66	85

(French Canadian) The subject is male, age 31-40. Parent of autistic child. *I had to resubmit the test once I had the chance to look at the French version. Regards, CC*

Diagnosis: NP type

The test shows Dominant NP type with a low S score (13). As would be expected for a highly perfectionistic personality type, the focus F score is >> 50. The temperament T and extroversion E scores are low (8, 56), again indicating a sociable, but reserved, individual.

The basic difference between the test results for NP and NPA− types (see the examples in Chap. 5) is the lower S scores in NP dominant types.

The subject in this Case is the parent of an autistic child. This issue is relevant here, as in our experience children with developmental disabilities who acquire diagnoses in the autistic spectrum (ASD) are most often NP types. More specifically, these young individuals frequently give NPA test results of "NP type with very high S score", or in our terminology "N− P

Borderline type" (see also Cases 26 and 27 in Chap. 6). This is in accordance with NPA genetics by which an NP child must have: 1) at least one parent who is an N or NP type, and 2) at least one parent who has the P trait. For a further discussion of the genetic mechanisms by which the NPA traits are transmitted, see Benis, 2017d.

7 NA type, aggressive... and into sadomasochism

3 3 4 4 0 4 3 2 2 3 0 4 1 4 4 4 4 4 0 1 4 1 0 1 0
0 0 0 4 4 0 2 2 0 4 1 0 4 3 3 0 3 3 0 4 0 4 4 2 3

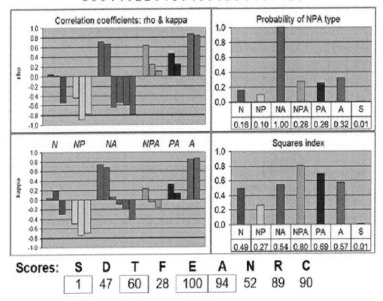

Scores:	S	D	T	F	E	A	N	R	C
	1	47	60	28	100	94	52	89	90

The subject is female, age 21-30. *I can be agressive, but agression tends to be very controlled and can be restricted to when necessary rather than uncontrolled; also I can be very focussed (company director) and also very analytical. Not particularly submissive. Only depressed if bored.* [the S score] *1 is a VERY low score, and honestly (shhh) lol even I get slightly anxious if there's something big I've got to do!* :) *interestingly, though dominant in life, I am into sadomasochism as both top and bottom, and have a preference for men who can outdominate me and reverse the everyday situation. Not yet found one* :(*lol Interesting test.*

Diagnosis: NA type

The test shows very low S score (1), low F score (28), and very high T and E scores (60, 100), consistent with a Dominant NA type. The A score is also very high (94). The N score is relatively low (52), but this is because of a poor correlation of the subject's answers with those of a non-aggressive N type, not because of inhibition of trait N. The very low F score is concordant with the non-perfectionism of the NA type.

This individual is no doubt a very extroverted, aggressive individual. Nevertheless, she hints at depression, boredom, and a lack of fulfillment in "playing the game" of dominance and submission. She claims to be very focused and analytical in her workplace, but the test suggests the opposite.

2 4 1 3 4 0 2 2 2 2 2 4 2 0 4 4 0 3 0 2 0 3 0 0 0
3 4 1 4 1 3 2 0 3 4 3 0 4 2 3 2 2 3 3 2 1 0 3 0 2

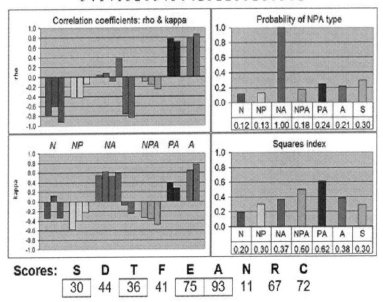

Scores:	S	D	T	F	E	A	N	R	C
	30	44	36	41	75	93	11	67	72

The subject is female, age 21-30. *Only agressive when someone does something disrespectful, otherwise i'm pretty chill or even kind ... But if somone wronged me or tried to dominate me (if they are family members i explode until they either crumble then pick them up or they take back what they said) i don't react at the time they disrespected me but that moment marks the begining of the end. I usually just mentally abuse them while keeping my perfect image (that way they are 100 pr cent sure it's all their fault) or give a very calm blow to their deepest insecurity...*

Diagnosis: NA type

The test shows low-moderate S score (30), low F score (41), and moderately high T and E scores (36, 75), consistent with a Dominant NA type. The A score is also very high (93). The N score is very low (11), but this is because of a poor correlation of the subject's answers with those of the "non-aggressive N type" reference test. The F score of < 50 is what one would expect with the non-perfectionism of the NA type.

The panel displaying the Squares indexes (lower right) illustrates how

NA types typically do not confine themselves to the NA category of questions, but rather answer positively to some in all of the categories.

The subject's comment illustrates some of the vindictive capacities of an aggressive Dominant NA personality type.

9 NPA+ type... or maybe a high-temperament NP type?

2 2 1 1 1 1 3 0 2 2 0 3 3 1 2 3 0 0 2 1 1 0 2 4 1
0 3 3 3 3 0 2 3 0 2 1 0 2 3 0 1 0 0 4 3 1 2 2 1 0

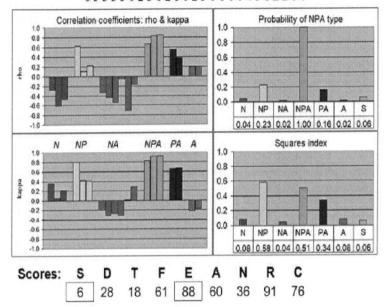

Scores:	S	D	T	F	E	A	N	R	C
	6	28	18	61	88	60	36	91	76

The subject is male, age 21-30. *I'm undecided between low temperament NPA and high temperament NP.*

Diagnosis: NPA+ type

The test shows very low S score (6), moderately high F score (61), moderate T score (18), and elevated E score (88), consistent with a Dominant NPA type. The A score is moderate (60). The N score is low (36), reflective of the bridling effect of the P trait on the N trait in the NPA+ character type.

The subject is unsure whether his type is "low temperament NPA" or "high temperament NP", and the test results are somewhat equivocal as well. The Squares index is higher for the NP category as compared to the NPA category, but the correlation coefficients were higher for NPA+ (orange bars) for both the rho and kappa functions. In addition, the elevated E score of 88 would be very unusual for an NP type. The test algorithm chose the NPA Dominant type unequivocally.

The moderate aggression A score of 60 is typical for the NPA+

Dominant type. Higher A scores in the range of 75-100 are found only in the non-perfectionistic Dominant A or NA types.

Note that we sometimes use the notation "NPA+ type" to differentiate the Dominant NPA character type from the generic term "NPA type".

4 0 2 4 0 0 4 0 4 4 0 3 2 0 0 2 2 4 4 3 0 2 0 4 0
4 4 0 1 0 0 1 4 4 2 0 0 0 3 0 1 0 0 0 4 2 0 0 4 0

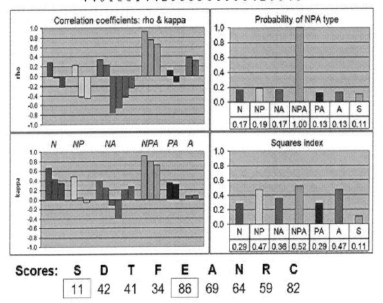

Scores:	S	D	T	F	E	A	N	R	C
	11	42	41	34	86	69	64	59	82

The subject is female, age 51-60. Explosive rages.

Diagnosis: NPA+ type

The test shows low S score (11), moderately low F score (34), moderately high T score (41), and elevated E score (86), consistent with a Dominant NPA type. The A score is moderately high (69). The N score is only moderate (64), reflective of the bridling effect of the P trait on the N trait in the NPA+ character type.

The correlation coefficients were the highest for the NPA category (orange bars) for both the rho and kappa functions. With the elevated E score of 86, the test algorithm chose the NPA Dominant type unequivocally.

With both traits N and A being fully expressed, the NPA+ Dominant type is especially vulnerable to uncontrollable "explosive rages" (see Fig. 3 of Chap. 1). In this combined "NA rage" there is a mass discharge of the autonomic nervous system causing the involuntary behavioral outburst. In individuals of light skin color, this is the classic red-faced, florid rage, sometimes likened to a "tantrum". In contrast, in the non-sanguine A and PA types, the pure "A rage" is associated with a mass discharge of the sympathetic nervous system and an associated pallid complexion in individuals of light skin color (see also Benis, 1985).

11 PA type with "N" Squares index of 0

0 4 0 3 0 0 3 0 3 4 1 3 1 0 4 3 1 2 4 3 0 0 0 0 0
1 3 0 4 4 1 0 3 0 4 0 1 4 0 0 0 0 2 4 1 0 4 0 0 3

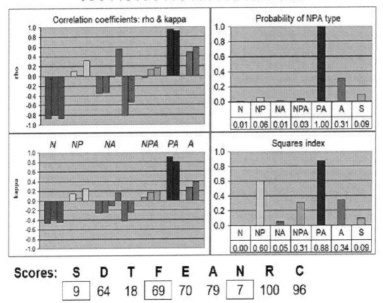

Scores: S   D   T   F   E   A   N   R   C
         9   64 18 69 70 79 7 100 96

(French version). The subject is male, age less than 21. *No particular pathology. Good test, one of the best that I have found on the web.*

« Pas de pathologie particulière. Bon test, un des meilleurs que j'ai trouvé sur le web. »

Diagnosis: PA type

The test shows very low S score (9), high F score (69), low T score (18), moderately high E score (70), and moderately high A score (79) consistent with a Dominant (non-sanguine) PA type. The N score is rock-bottom (7) characteristic of a non-sanguine type.

Note the Squares index of 0 for the N category, meaning that the subject answered with a "0" to all seven questions in this category. In fact, the N and PA character types are mirror images of each other, in the sense that neither has any of the NPA traits of the other. Very often, we find that N types show disdain for the questions of the PA category, and vice versa. This antipathy also shows itself in the very negative rho and kappa correlation coefficients in the N group in the graphs above.

One may have noticed that the Squares index for the NP category is relatively high in this Case (0.60), but the low rho and kappa values in the NP group, and the relatively high E and A scores would rule out the diagnosis of Dominant NP type for this young man.

1 3 0 1 1 1 2 0 3 3 1 0 1 0 3 0 0 0 3 0 2 0 0 0 0
0 1 2 2 2 2 0 2 0 1 1 1 2 0 0 0 0 1 1 0 1 4 0 0 0

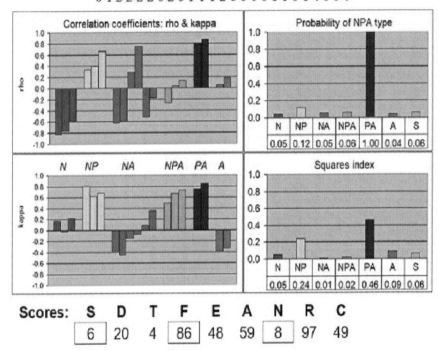

Scores:

S	D	T	F	E	A	N	R	C
6	20	4	86	48	59	8	97	49

The subject is male, age 21-30. *Some parts of the PA caricature are accurate. My grandmother had Paranoid schizophrenia, and my uncle was diagnosed with Paranoid PD* [Personality Disorder].

Diagnosis: PA type

The test shows Dominant (non-sanguine) PA type with very low S score (6). As would be expected for a highly perfectionistic personality type, the focus F score of 86 is >> 50. The temperament T and extroversion E scores are low (4, 48), indicating a Dominant, but reserved, individual.

The subject in this Case has a family history of both paranoid personality disorder and paranoid schizophrenia. This family history is relevant here for three reasons:

First, the PA character type is especially prone to paranoia, sometimes of pathological proportions.

Second, in comparison to the NPA+ type, the PA type has a relatively high risk of schizophrenia, and in particular, of paranoid schizophrenia. In the NPA model, types having only one trait, A or N, are at higher risk.

Third, in accordance with NPA genetics, non-sanguine types cluster in families. In particular, a PA child must have at least one parent who is a non-sanguine A or PA type. For a further discussion of the genetic mechanisms by which the NPA traits are transmitted, see Benis, 2017d.

2 3 1 2 1 2 2 0 4 4 0 4 0 0 4 1 3 4 3 1 2 0 0 2 0
0 0 0 4 0 0 2 0 0 1 0 0 4 0 0 3 4 4 0 2 0 0 0 0 4

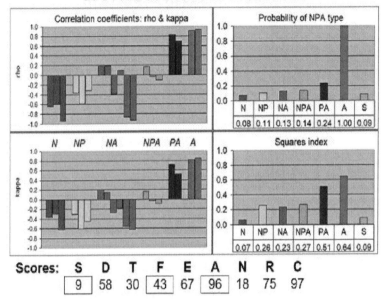

Scores:	S	D	T	F	E	A	N	R	C
	9	58	30	43	67	96	18	75	97

The subject is male, age 31-40.

Diagnosis: A type

The test shows Dominant (non-sanguine) A type with very low S score (9). As would be expected for a non-perfectionistic personality type, the focus F score of 43 is < 50. The temperament T and extroversion E scores are moderate (30, 67), indicating a Dominant, outgoing individual. The N score is very low (18) characteristic of a non-sanguine type. As expected, the A score of 96 is close to the maximum value.

Like the N and PA types, the A and NP types are mirror images, in the sense that neither type has any of the NPA traits of the other. There is often an aversion of the A type to questions in the NP category, and vice versa. In this case, this aversion is reflected in the highly negative rho and kappa correlation coefficients in the NP group.

In sum, the present test is the classical response of the Dominant non-sanguine, aggressive A type. Very low S score is typical, as if the A type had a disdain for the questions in the S category. In contrast, A types also frequently have a liking for the questions in the (non-sanguine) PA category, so there is sometimes an overlap between the A and PA diagnostic categories (see the next Case).

4 2 3 0 0 0 1 0 4 3 0 3 3 2 3 3 1 4 2 4 1 2 0 2 0
3 3 1 4 4 1 1 0 1 0 3 2 4 1 0 2 3 0 4 1 1 4 0 1 2

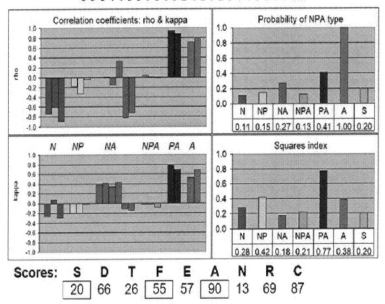

Scores:	S	D	T	F	E	A	N	R	C
	20	66	26	55	57	90	13	69	87

(Russian version; location: Western Russia). The subject is male, age 21-30. Rage disorder (приступы ярости).

Diagnosis: A type

The test shows Dominant (non-sanguine) A type with low S score (20). The focus F score (55), or slightly high for a non-perfectionistic A type. The temperament T and extroversion E scores are moderate (26, 57), indicating a Dominant, outgoing individual. The N score is very low (13) characteristic of a non-sanguine type. As expected, the A score of 90 is very high.

This case shows a very high response to questions in the PA category (Squares index graph, above). This is reflected in the somewhat elevated F score and in the very high rho and kappa correlation coefficients in the PA group. Nevertheless, given the very high A score, the test algorithm chose Dominant A type, rather than PA type.

Of interest is that this test comes from Western Russia, which we had previously identified as an "Authoritarian habitancy" (a region having a high prevalence of non-sanguine A and PA types). Interestingly, non-sanguine A and PA types are concentrated only in the regions of Eastern Europe/Russia, the Balkans and the Middle East. For further discussion of the geographic distribution of the NPA traits, see Benis, 2017a.

15 A type with potential for sadistic vindictiveness

2 4 2 3 0 0 3 0 4 3 0 3 2 1 3 3 3 4 1 1 4 1 0 3 1
0 4 0 3 4 1 2 3 1 1 0 0 4 3 0 2 1 0 0 3 2 3 0 3 4

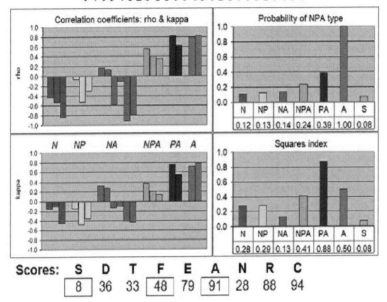

Scores:

S	D	T	F	E	A	N	R	C
8	36	33	48	79	91	28	88	94

The subject is male, age under 21. *I will admit that i have a dominant agrressive personality, but i lack the arrogance that is associated with this personality. I have no desire to be better than everyone. I am often quick to take resposibilty for my own faults and actions. In a fit of rage, I become sadistic in my actions and my thought process. As it stands i do not place alot of value in humanity, so if crossed by someone i allowed to become close to me, worst case scenarios are likely to become a reality.*

Diagnosis: A type

The test indicates Dominant (non-sanguine) A type with very low S score (8). As would be expected for a non-perfectionistic personality type, the focus F score of 48 is < 50. The temperament T and extroversion E scores are high-moderate (33, 79), indicating a Dominant, outgoing individual. The N score is very low (28) characteristic of a non-sanguine type. As expected, the A score of 91 is close to the maximum value.

Both this test and that of the previous Case indicate a rage disorder, which for an A type would be the classic pallid-faced aggressive-vindictive

"A rage" (Fig. 3 of Chap. 1). In the present test, the subject's comments are equivocal. On the one hand, he wishes to be a responsible member of society. But on the other hand, he is proud of his aggressive-sadistic potential, and he seems waiting for the opportunity for the "worst case scenario to become a reality".

CHAPTER 5

Passive aggressive types

NA– NA=

NPA– NPA=

1 0 3 0 0 0 3 3 3 0 1 4 4 4 2 3 1 0 3 4 4 0 3 3 3
4 2 0 4 3 3 3 1 4 0 3 3 3 3 3 3 0 0 0 3 4 2 3 3 0

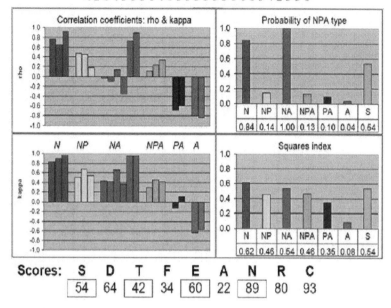

Scores:

S	D	T	F	E	A	N	R	C
54	64	42	34	60	22	89	80	93

The subject is female, age 31- 40. Fibromyalgia. *I think it is pretty accurate. I have a degenerative spine disease, arthritis, and fibromyalgia. There are also several family members diagnosed with bipolar. I was always taught to control my temper so I do have a lot of pent up anger that explodes when I am alone and then turns to tears. I was told kids are to be seen and not heard and am just now starting to come out of my shell.*

Diagnosis: NA− type (or, N or NA type with high S score)

The test is consistent with NA− (non-compliant) Passive aggressive type with moderately high S score (54), moderately high T and E scores (42, 60), low F score (34), low A score (22) and high N score (89).

On the NPA test, the NA− type is differentiated from the NA Dominant type mainly by the higher S score of > 40 in the NA− type. However, the Test generally cannot differentiate between "NA− type" and "N or NA type with high S score", so the latter would be alternative diagnoses.

The low F score (< 50) and the low correlation coefficients for the NP category differentiate this test from the perfectionistic Passive aggressive types (NPA−, NPA=). Although the detachment D score is somewhat high in this test (64), the elevated T and N scores suggest that the subject is basically a sociable, active individual.

2 0 3 3 0 3 1 0 0 2 3 0 2 1 0 3 0 0 0 3 2 2 1 2 0
3 1 0 2 3 3 0 1 0 3 2 3 0 0 0 2 0 0 2 3 4 1 0 1 0

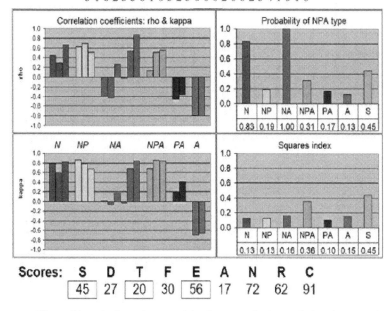

Probability of NPA type						
N	NP	NA	NPA	PA	A	S
0.83	0.19	1.00	0.31	0.17	0.13	0.45

Squares index						
N	NP	NA	NPA	PA	A	S
0.13	0.13	0.16	0.36	0.10	0.15	0.45

Scores:	S	D	T	F	E	A	N	R	C
	45	27	20	30	56	17	72	62	91

The subject is female, age 41-50. Myopia (nearsighted, severe). *Pretty accurate. I feel I have a tendency toward aggression and I have a tendency toward anxiety/fear and I like to be funny/well-liked and I can be very concerned with how i look, physically, but I have learned to deal with all of these better and to see appropriateness or inappropriateness in my behaviors and I tend to get a long with almost anyone. I tend to be a "fence-sitter" I see the good or positives in both sides of the equation, i.e. Republican/Democrat, liberal/conservative*

Diagnosis: NA– type (or, N or NA type with high S score)

The test is most consistent with NA– Passive aggressive type with moderately high S score (45), moderate T and E scores (20, 56), low F score (30), low A score (17) and moderate N score (72).

As in the preceding case, the test cannot differentiate between "NA–type" and "N or NA type with elevated S score", so the latter would be alternative diagnoses.

The moderately high S score indicates NA– type, rather than the (compliant) Passive aggressive types NA=, who generally have very high S scores (> 75).

The more moderate T, E and N scores suggest that this subject is a less extroverted individual than in the preceding case.

3 2 3 2 4 0 2 3 2 1 4 2 1 2 2 0 2 1 3 4 0 1 4 2 3
3 2 1 2 2 4 2 2 3 2 1 4 0 1 4 4 2 2 1 0 4 1 1 1 1

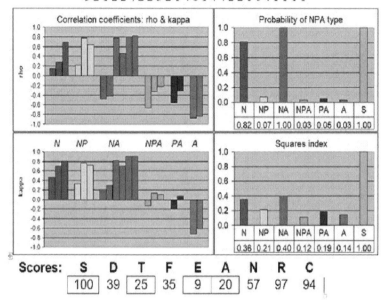

Scores:

S	D	T	F	E	A	N	R	C
100	39	25	35	9	20	57	97	94

The subject is female, age 31-40. Depression, on medication. *Lifelong extreme shyness, depression, possible covert narcissism, I am very submissive around most people but have huge amounts of anger and aggression in me that most people would never guess is there, except for my close family/spouse who see a different me altogether.*

Diagnosis: NA= type

The test indicates (compliant) Passive aggressive NA= type with the maximum possible S score (100), moderate T score (25), very low E score (9), very low A score (20), and low F score (35). The N score is moderate (57).

In general, the NA= type is differentiated from the NA– type mainly by the higher S score (> 75) in the NA= type. This test might also be consistent with an N or NA type with very high S score, but given the subject's comments regarding her shyness, that would be less likely.

Commonly reported by subjects who give test results of "NA= type" are:

inability to focus, lack of self-confidence, covert narcissism, lifelong extreme shyness, depression, panic attacks, borderline type, worrying about appearance, avoiding confrontation with others and *"free-floating"* anxiety. Often the comments are somewhat disordered, and lack proper capitalization and punctuation, hinting at the absence of the P trait.

19 NA= type with inability to focus

1 1 2 2 3 1 1 1 1 0 4 2 0 4 1 0 0 1 2 4 2 0 3 0 0
0 2 0 2 0 4 1 3 3 2 1 4 2 4 0 3 0 0 2 2 4 0 1 3 0

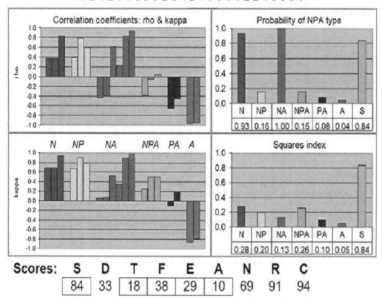

Scores:

S	D	T	F	E	A	N	R	C
84	33	18	38	29	10	69	91	94

The subject is female, age 41-50. *Unable to focus, lack of self confidence. lack of organization. i have no clue how to get my life in order. out of control. i have trouble finding humor in things that should be funny. sometimes it easier to just stare into space with a mind that is empty or not really thinking of anything. when i get my bills out to pay i can't concentrate on what to first and get aggrivated and give up until they call. sometimes my mind is on overload and i can't focus on one for focusing on 20. i guess the rages are from all of the lack of being in control and watching my life go to the pot and theres nothing i can do to stop it. and in the meantime ruining my marriage and home because now i'm a b---ch.*

Diagnosis: NA= type

The test indicates (compliant) Passive aggressive NA= type with very high S score (84), low T score (18), low E score (29), very low A score (10), and low F score (38). The N score is moderate (69).

With the very high S score and low F score, the test is very similar to the preceding one, and the subject's non-perfectionistic comments are consistent with an NA= type.

2 1 0 1 3 2 3 0 2 3 3 4 4 2 3 3 0 2 3 4 0 0 2 1 1
0 1 0 4 3 1 3 0 2 4 4 4 1 3 0 2 2 0 4 0 1 3 0 1 1

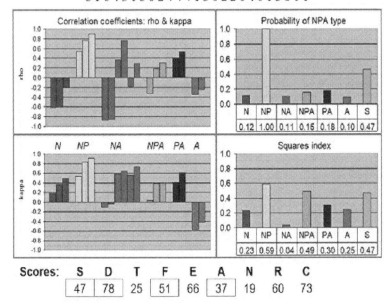

Scores:

S	D	T	F	E	A	N	R	C
47	78	25	51	66	37	19	60	73

(French version) The subject is male, age 21-30. Migraines. *The results given here seems to me correct, I also have difficulties in social relations in general. I tend to be very sensitive and easily believe that I'm being taken for a fool or mocked. I can overreact to someone who raises his voice or who has bad manners, I have had several times violent verbal exchanges with complete strangers because they had shown me lack of respect. I am also very resentful and never forgive the least offense. Basically, I am not an aggressive person but I feel that I have to pretend to be so to have a minimum of consideration. Most of the time my aggressive reactions result more from a calculation ("I must react, otherwise I will pass for a weakling") than from a real impulse...*

Diagnosis: NPA− type

The test indicates (non-compliant) Passive aggressive NPA− type with a moderately elevated S score (47), moderate T and E scores (25, 66), moderate F score (51), and low A score (37). The N score is also low (19).

Higher F scores and lower N scores help to differentiate NPA− types from their NA− cousins. In this case, the D score is also elevated (78), indicating a tendency to detachment from social relations. However, the main impression from the subject's comment is an active, perfectionistic individual who has the A− trait of inhibited aggression.

21 NPA– type in abusive relationship

0 0 3 0 0 0 2 0 3 1 4 2 2 0 0 2 0 0 4 2 2 0 4 0 1
3 0 0 4 3 4 0 0 2 3 3 4 0 0 0 3 0 0 2 3 3 0 0 1 0

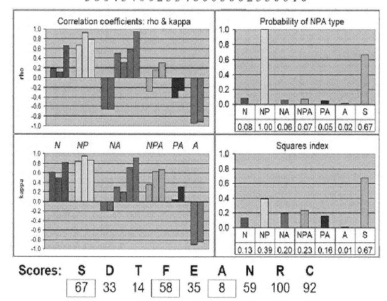

Scores:	S	D	T	F	E	A	N	R	C
	67	33	14	58	35	8	59	100	92

The subject is female, age 31-40. Asthma. *I am recovering from an abusive relationship with an aggressive narcissistic type, I am not narcisstic myself but may show traits until I can heal myself."*

Diagnosis: NPA– type (or possibly NPA= type)

The test indicates Passive aggressive NPA– or NPA= type with a high S score (67), and low T (14), E (35) and A (8) scores. The F score (58) is greater than 50, or in the range that indicates the presence of P trait.

As exemplified by the subject's comment, the NPA– type (or NPA= type) is often attracted to a Dominant NA type, where an unbalanced relationship based on dominance and submission (and sometimes overt sadomasochism) ensues. Although the dependent partner in this case is female, in such relationships of dominance and submission, the dependent partner may be either male or female, and the relationship needs not be a heterosexual one.

A classic presentation of relationships of dominance-submission based on the trait of aggression was published by psychiatrist Karen Horney (1954), who termed such bonds "morbid dependency". Although the NPA– and Dominant NA pairing is the classic one, such abusive relationships can readily occur with either partner being an A, NA, PA, NPA or even a Passive aggressive type, as well.

1 3 0 2 4 0 0 3 4 4 4 2 3 0 4 1 0 0 4 3 0 0 3 1 0
2 2 2 4 3 3 1 4 3 0 3 4 3 3 0 4 1 2 4 1 4 4 0 2 0

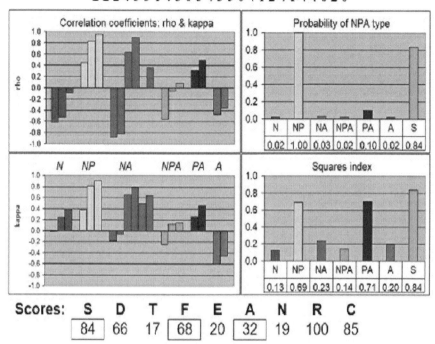

Scores:	S	D	T	F	E	A	N	R	C
	84	66	17	68	20	32	19	100	85

The subject is male, age 31-40. *The NA descriptions don't match at all, the whole NPA– page seems "right", but also the short NA– description sounded right on the NA page. I have strong camera fobia unless it's a mass-photo like a school class. I prefer to be in groups size of 2-3, get minor anxiety being near a large group even if they're relatives/friends. And I'm from Finland. I've not been diagnosed but I have watched TV programs about asp/autism and much of it seems familiar. I think everything must be in perfect order but I don't feel like having energy to do things perfectly, I do expect perfection from others quite "naturally".*

Diagnosis: NPA= type (or possibly Borderline N– P type)

The subject's test and comments are most consistent with the perfectionistic (compliant) Passive aggressive NPA= type, with a very high S score (84), and low T, E, A and N scores (17, 20, 32, 19). The F score being greater than 50 is consistent with the presence of the P trait.

The subject's comments regarding social anxiety and having a "camera phobia" are common in types having the A− or A= trait. Interestingly, the subject is from Finland, which we had previously identified as an "Introspective habitancy" (a region having a high prevalence of A− or A= trait). For further discussion of the geographic distribution of the NPA traits, see our monograph (Benis, 2017a).

CHAPTER 6

Resigned types
N –A NP –A

3 1 0 1 3 0 3 0 3 3 3 4 4 0 3 3 0 1 4 4 0 0 2 2 0
0 1 0 4 4 2 3 0 1 4 3 3 1 3 0 2 0 0 4 0 2 4 0 0 1

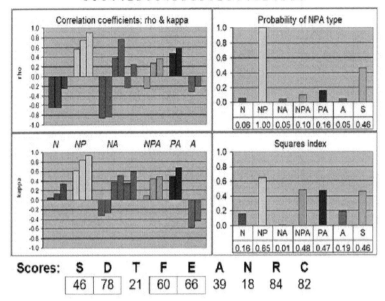

Scores:	S	D	T	F	E	A	N	R	C
	46	78	21	60	66	39	18	84	82

The subject is male, age 21-30. *Interesting. I've read the personality types descriptions and I find more of myself in your "resigned types". Because of this I was surprised scoring so high in the E scale: I can't bear social gatherings and I rather stay reserved in social situations to avoid being too much bothered by others.*

Diagnosis: Resigned type NP –A (former NPA– type)

The test shows NP type with moderate S score (46) and high detachment D score (78), so the diagnosis is consistent with the comment in which the subject identifies with "Resigned types". Before becoming a Resigned type, the subject was likely a Passive aggressive NPA– type in adolescence, as indicated by the moderately high S score.

The F score of >50 is consistent with the presence of the P trait in the character type.

Despite the subject's comment, the E score of 66 is in the mid-range, and not particularly high.

24 Resigned type NP −A with "Peter Pan syndrome"

1 1 0 0 3 0 3 0 3 2 3 3 4 0 3 2 0 2 3 4 0 0 2 2 1
4 1 0 4 3 2 3 0 3 4 4 4 1 3 0 2 0 0 4 0 2 3 0 0 0

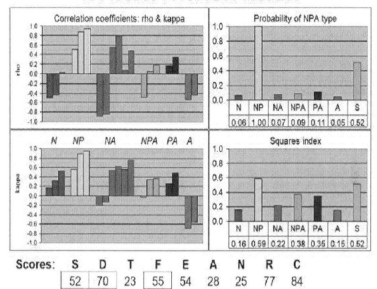

Scores:	S	D	T	F	E	A	N	R	C
	52	70	23	55	54	28	25	77	84

(French version) The subject is male, age 21-30. *Recently diagnosed as having Peter Pan syndrome because I refuse to relate to adult social life and prefer to devote myself to solitary hobbies. My superiors and colleagues have difficulty managing me because I do not tolerate authority or criticism. I do not look for the company of women and sexuality because I find it too difficult to manage, which worries my entourage. This test is interesting because yes I think to be perfectionistic: I find the world too imperfect and others too unpredictable so I prefer to stay in my own world that fits me better...*

Diagnosis: Resigned type NP −A (former NPA− type)

The test shows a moderately high S score (52) and a high Detachment score (70), so the diagnosis is consistent with the comment in which the subject identifies with a solitary life-style and the avoidance of social contact. Note the similarity of this test to the preceding one.

The F score of >50 and the comment regarding being "perfectionistic" are consistent with the presence of the P trait in the character type.

Note: "Peter Pan syndrome describes one's inability to believe that they are of an older age or to engage in behaviour usually associated with adulthood" [*Wikipedia*].

25 Resigned type N –A (or Detached type –N)

3 1 3 1 2 0 1 0 3 3 3 2 2 4 4 3 1 1 4 3 3 0 3 3 3
1 2 0 4 4 2 4 0 1 4 4 3 3 3 0 2 1 0 3 1 2 3 0 4 0

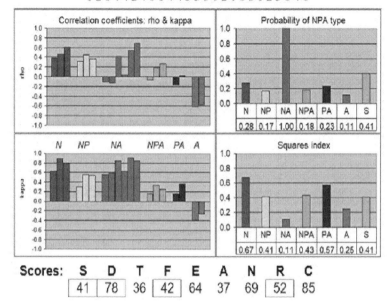

Scores:	S	D	T	F	E	A	N	R	C
	41	78	36	42	64	37	69	52	85

(French version) The subject is male, age 31-40. *Your theory is very interesting. I do not recognize myself at all in the NA character described here, but I have never encountered such an accurate description of my life as in the "resigned type". To have few desires, especially those involving other people, is the best way to not be frustrated and therefore de facto to be at peace.*

Diagnosis: Resigned type N –A (or Detached type –N)

At first glance, tests appears to show "NA type" with a moderate S score (41), so the diagnosis here comes from the elevated D score (78) and the comment in which the subject identifies with "Resigned types".

The F score of < 50 is consistent with the lack of the P trait in the character type. The moderate S score indicates that before adopting a life-style of resignation, the subject was formerly a Dominant N or NA type, or a Passive aggressive NA– type. If he was a Dominant N type, his NPA designation now would be: non-aggressive Detached type, –N.

The low R score indicates that the subject's answers did not correlate well with any of the 19 Standard tests. A low R score ("coherence") can occur if the subject responds in an unusual or exceptional manner. Here, the subject responded in an "exceptional" manner, since none of the 19 Standard tests fits the profile of a Resigned type with a high D score.

CHAPTER 7

Borderline types

–N

N–P

P–A

–A

1 1 0 0 4 0 3 2 1 0 3 0 4 0 2 0 0 0 3 4 0 0 4 0 0

0 0 1 4 3 4 0 3 0 0 3 4 0 0 0 4 0 0 4 0 4 1 0 0 0

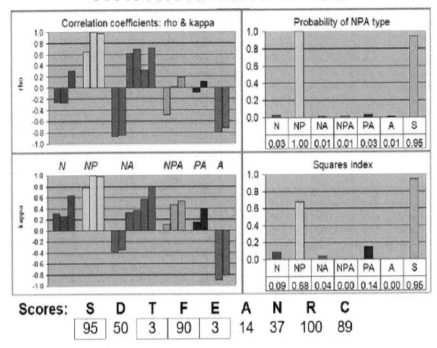

Scores:
S	D	T	F	E	A	N	R	C
95	50	3	90	3	14	37	100	89

The subject is male, age 31-40. ADD, Asperger's. *Sounds accurate. I have OCD and am diagnosed with ADD (inattentive subtype), self-diagnosed with Asperger's. I am male-assigned at birth, but deep down feel like a girl and seem to be trans.*

Borderline N– P type

The test shows "NP type" with very high S score (95), very high F score (90) and very low T, E and A scores (3, 3, 14). In the context of autism/Asperger syndrome, this would be the Borderline N– P type.

The NPA test cannot differentiate between the Borderline N– P type and NPA= type (see Case #22, above), so it is the autism/Asperger syndrome diagnosis, together with the very high S score, that makes the diagnosis of Borderline N– P type here.

The N– P type is typically a non-aggressive, socially aloof, perfectionistic individual. The N trait, although present in the N– P type, is inhibited. Thus, the sociability, smiling and outgoing nature of the N type is doubly suppressed in the N– P type by 1) the P trait and 2) genetic inhibition of the N trait. (The "–" sign *following* N in "N– P" indicates genetic inhibition expressing itself with juvenile onset. A "–" sign *preceding* N, as in "–NP" would designate a Dominant NP type who became a socially withdrawn Borderline/detached type after maturity.)

0 2 0 0 4 0 0 0 0 0 4 0 2 0 2 0 0 0 4 4 0 0 4 0 2
0 2 3 4 3 4 0 2 0 1 0 4 0 0 0 4 0 0 3 0 4 4 0 0 0

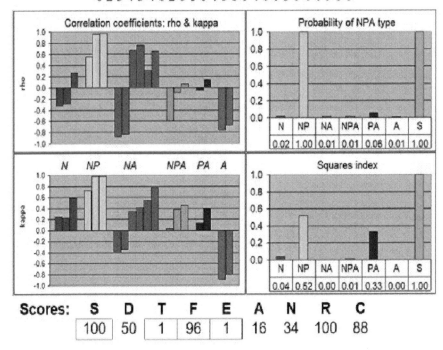

Scores:	**S**	**D**	**T**	**F**	**E**	**A**	**N**	**R**	**C**
	100	50	1	96	1	16	34	100	88

(French version) The subject is male, age under 21, reporting BPD, or borderline personality disorder. *Maybe I am extremely gifted and/or Asperger syndrome*

« Peut être suis je surdoué et/ou asperger. »

Diagnosis: Borderline N– P type

As in the preceding case, the test shows NP type with very high S score (the maximum of 100), very high F score (96) and extremely low T, E and A scores (1, 1, 16). In the context of autism/Asperger syndrome and the reported BPD, this would be our Borderline N– P type.

Note the striking similarity in results in this and the preceding case, given that the two individuals are of different age, come from different cultures and took different language versions of the test.

In our experience, extremely gifted young people, including the classical "autistic savant", are often perfectionistic NP (or N– P Borderline) types who have an autistic spectrum disorder, or ASD.

2 4 0 2 0 0 0 0 1 4 0 4 3 0 2 2 0 3 4 4 2 0 0 0 0
0 4 1 4 4 4 0 0 0 0 0 0 4 0 0 3 0 0 2 0 1 4 3 0 0

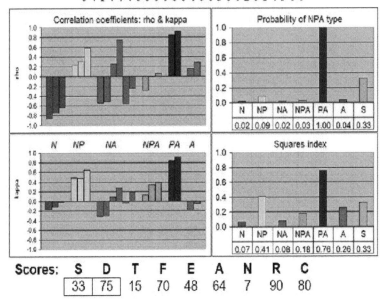

Scores:	S	D	T	F	E	A	N	R	C
	33	75	15	70	48	64	7	90	80

The subject is male, age under 21. Migraine headaches. *I know what I can do is evil, but I carry on, because I enjoy being evil, I enjoy people's suffer.*

Diagnosis: Detached Borderline type P –A

The test shows a (non-sanguine) PA type with moderately elevated S score (33) and a high Detachment D score (75). The diagnosis is consistent with the subject's antisocial comment in which he identifies with sadistic schemes rather than with conventional social behavior.

The moderate T, E and A scores (15, 48, 64) indicate a medium temperament individual with somewhat inhibited aggression.

The elevated F score (70) indicates a character type having trait P.

The very low N score (7) is what one would expect for a non-sanguine type.

Since the S score is only modestly elevated, this individual could be a genetically Dominant PA type, who is adopting a life style of detached inhibited aggression due to his particular environmental constraints.

Note that the P –A type also falls into the category of "Resigned types". However, the non-sanguine –A and P –A types have neither fully expressed N nor A trait, so they are better discussed in our classification as "Borderline types".

2 4 0 2 0 0 0 4 4 4 0 4 3 0 4 2 0 3 0 4 4 4 0 0 0
0 4 0 4 4 3 0 0 0 2 0 2 4 0 0 4 4 0 4 0 0 4 0 0 4

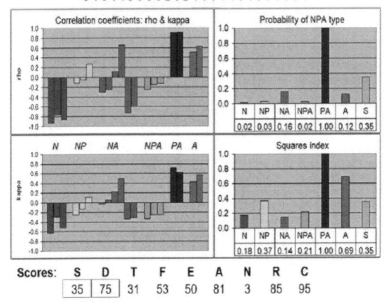

Scores:	S	D	T	F	E	A	N	R	C
	35	75	31	53	50	81	3	85	95

(Russian version) The subject is male, aged under 21. *Is the test accurate? Surprisingly, yes. For example, if I have a desire to kill someone or hit someone, then I usually hold back, or rather I always hold back. Afterward, either I just suck it up, or I become even more embittered with everyday life.*

("На удивление да. Например если у меня есть желание кого нибудь убить или ударить, то я обычно сдерживаюсь, а точнее всегда сдерживаюсь. После либо матерю воздух, либо становлюсь ещё более озлобленным в повседневной жизни.")

Diagnosis: Detached Borderline type P –A

Very similar to the preceding case, this test indicates a (non-sanguine) PA type with moderately high S score (35) and a high Detachment D score (75). As in the preceding case, the diagnosis is consistent with the antisocial comment in which the subject identifies with aggressive-sadistic behavior rather than with conventional mores.

Compared to the preceding case, the more elevated T and A scores indicate an individual with higher temperament.

Again, this individual could be a genetically Dominant PA type, who is adopting a life style of detached inhibited aggression due to environmental constraints.

3 4 4 4 1 4 2 0 4 4 0 4 4 0 2 4 0 2 0 4 2 2 0 4 0
1 3 1 4 3 0 0 2 0 4 1 0 3 0 2 0 4 4 4 1 0 4 2 4 4

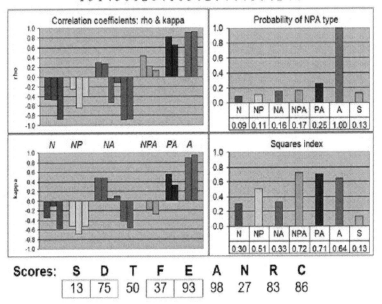

Scores:

S	D	T	F	E	A	N	R	C
13	75	50	37	93	98	27	83	86

The subject is male, age 31-40. LGBT. *Trained Musician (hobby/ death metal), Licensed Pro (Judiciary/ double life), Lives alone since 20, very attractive physically, Confused about his gender, avoids sex, dislikes people, loves animals, nightmarish childhood, hopes it helps, loves science and reason.*

Diagnosis: Detached Borderline type –A

The test shows a (non-sanguine) A type with a very low S score (13) and a high Detachment D score (75). The diagnosis is consistent with the comment in which the subject identifies with social avoidance rather than with conventional social behavior.

The very high T, E and A scores indicate a high temperament individual with high innate aggression.

Since the S score is very low, this individual is likely a former Dominant A type, who is adopting a life style of detached inhibited aggression due to environmental constraints.

The −A type is a "Borderline type" because neither trait N nor A is fully expressed. The more common (sanguine) N −A and NP −A Resigned types are not Borderline types because they have fully expressed N trait. They are socially detached as well, but since they have fully expressed N trait, they generally have a lower risk of sociopathy or psychosis.

0 4 0 4 2 0 2 0 4 4 0 1 2 0 4 4 3 4 2 4 1 4 1 1 0
0 2 1 4 4 1 3 4 0 3 1 1 2 0 0 3 4 3 2 2 2 4 2 2 3

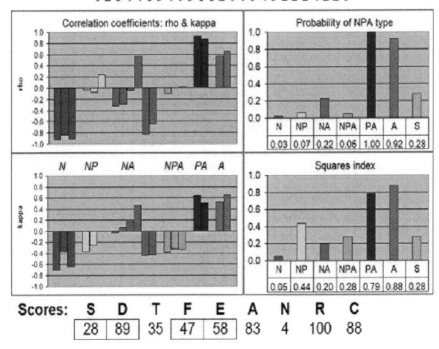

Scores:	S	D	T	F	E	A	N	R	C
	28	89	35	47	58	83	4	100	88

The subject is male, age 41-50. *major depression, anti-social, debilitated and behavior modified while in prison for 12 years.*

Diagnosis: Detached Borderline type –A (or possibly P –A)

The test shows a (non-sanguine) A or PA type with a low S score (28) and a high Detachment D score (89). The diagnosis is consistent with the comment in which the subject identifies with depression and antisocial avoidance rather than with conventional social behavior.

In comparison with the similar preceding case, the more moderate T, E and A scores indicate an individual of lower temperament. Here, the higher F score and higher correlation coefficients for PA type may indicate the presence of trait P, i.e., the alternative diagnosis of P –A type.

Since the S score is only modestly elevated, this individual could be a former Dominant A or PA type, who is adopting a life style of detached inhibited aggression due to very severe environmental constraints that he faced, which included incarceration in prison.

Both individuals in the last two cases — despite the harsh life pressures during adolescence — answered the questions of the test as if they were still Dominant A types. Despite becoming "resigned" to their life changes, deep in the character of these individuals remains the dominant trait of aggression... and that is how they responded on the Test.

4 1 1 0 1 2 0 1 1 1 0 2 3 3 2 3 1 1 2 0 4 1 1 1 1
0 0 0 1 1 1 1 0 0 0 1 0 2 1 1 0 1 0 1 1 0 1 1 3 0

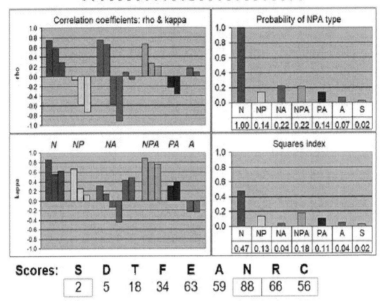

Scores: S D T F E A N R C
         2 5 18 34 63 59 88 66 56

The subject is male, age under 21. Schizophrenia. *How could I know if it was accurate. It was a bit silly. I'm a passive agressive empathic narcsissistic sociopath with paranoid schizophrenia. :-) and still I manage to be happier than most of the people in the world. Maybe evrybody needs a tiny bit more crazy in their life to enjoy the insanity that is life and the world. (Yes I know, that went a little deep maybe even psychotic/ delusonal sounding but hell if I know; I'm crazy!) thx for the test, it was kinda boring... but the fact that I like talking about myself and answering questions about myself helped me not to close this site. It wad nice!*

Diagnosis: Borderline N– type

The test shows N type with a very low S score of 2. The T and E scores (18, 63) are moderate. Here, the diagnosis of "Borderline, non-aggressive withdrawn type N–" comes from the subject's diagnosis of schizophrenia (SCZ). Most likely, this individual before becoming ill (the so-called "premorbid NPA personality type") was a Dominant N type.

The test results, in fact, are very similar to those commonly seen in the

Dominant N type (Chapter 4). The detachment D score is low (5). Unexpectedly, in our series of 92 subjects reporting the diagnosis of SCZ, only 10 had D scores >70, as if these subjects answered the questions of the test as healthy individuals, before becoming mentally ill.

CHAPTER 8

Other tests

33 Random answers to test and the R score

2 1 2 1 4 2 0 2 0 0 4 1 4 2 4 1 0 0 0 2 2 3 0 3 0
2 2 1 1 1 0 3 3 0 1 4 0 3 4 4 2 3 0 3 4 3 0 0 2 0

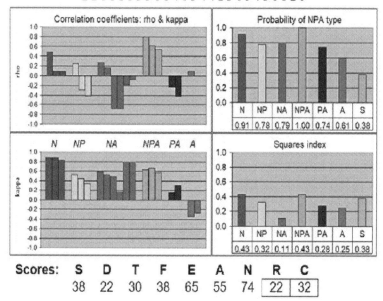

Scores:	S	D	T	F	E	A	N	R	C
	38	22	30	38	65	55	74	22	32

In this test, 50 random numbers from 0 to 4 were entered. The results for the Squares indexes, the correlation coefficients and the various test scores do not show any coherent pattern towards an NPA diagnosis. In particular, the C score (32) for statistical consistency between the rho and kappa functions is especially poor.

Values of the correlation coefficient r between the subject's answers and those of the 19 Standard tests are displayed in the figure below:

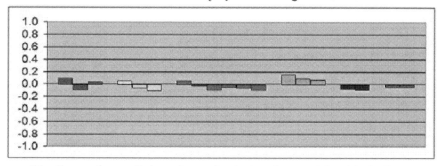

The figure shows all the values of r clustered around 0, with the largest value of r being equal to +0.15. As the *R score* ("for coherence") is calculated as the largest value of r plus its standard deviation, normalized to a scale of 100, R is here $(0.15 + 0.07) \times 100 = 22$, which is very low. In general, in the NPA test a value of $R < 50$ indicates poor or "exceptional" agreement with the Standard tests on which the test is based. Besides "randomness", there are many other possible reasons for a low R score giving an apparent incoherent response (see *Appendix A*).

3 0 3 2 0 3 1 0 0 0 0 0 0 4 0 4 3 0 0 4 4 0 3 1 3

0 0 0 3 0 1 1 0 1 0 4 4 0 3 3 1 0 0 3 3 3 0 3 4 0

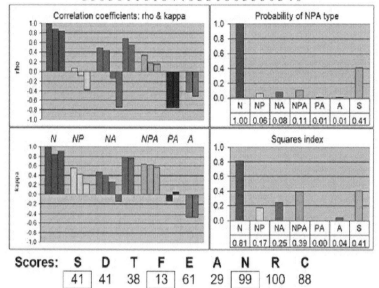

Scores:	S	D	T	F	E	A	N	R	C
	41	41	38	13	61	29	99	100	88

The subject is female, age 21-30. *I have cerebral palsy and move in a wheel-chair.*

Diagnosis: N type

The test is most consistent with Dominant N type having a moderately high S score (41), moderate T and E scores (38, 61), very low F score (13), and low A score (29). The N score (99) is close to the maximum, indicating almost perfect correlation with the N1 Standard reference test.

However, in general, the test cannot differentiate between "N type with elevated S score" and "NA− type", so the latter would be alternative diagnosis.

Cerebral palsy pertains to a group of "motor" or movement disorders that appear in early childhood. Often the disability is severe, and the patient is confined to a wheelchair during social interactions. Nevertheless, other than the moderately increased S score, the test results of this case do not show anything unusual and are in the normal ranges of those of a sociable individual.

3 2 3 3 1 1 2 0 2 2 1 3 2 1 2 3 2 0 1 0 2 0 1 2 2
0 1 2 1 4 1 2 2 1 1 0 2 2 3 2 2 0 0 3 3 3 3 3 1 0

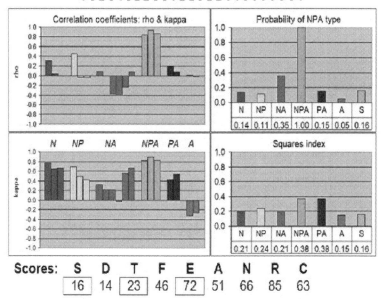

Scores:	S	D	T	F	E	A	N	R	C
	16	14	23	46	72	51	66	85	63

The subject is female, age 21-30. *I am* MBTI: ESTJ.

Diagnosis: NPA+ type

The test shows low S score (16), moderate F score (46), moderate T score (23), and elevated E score (72), consistent with a Dominant NPA+ type. The A score is moderate (51). The N score is only moderate (66), reflective of the bridling effect of the P trait on the N trait. With neither of the T, E or A scores showing extreme values, the test suggests an NPA+ individual who is able to keep the three fully-expressed traits in balance.

In the Myers-Briggs Type Indicator, or MBTI test, an Executive (ESTJ) "is someone with the Extraverted, Observant, Thinking, and Judging personality traits. They possess great fortitude, emphatically following their own sensible judgment. They often serve as a stabilizing force among others, able to offer solid direction amid adversity" [from www.16personalities.com].

The descriptions of the Myer Briggs ESTJ type are most consistent with our NPA Dominant type, so agreement between the two makes sense. However, with the 16 types in the MBTI system, quite obviously there cannot be an easy one-to-one comparison between the two systems. The NPA trait model, being biologically based on genetic loci, proposes to be the kind of standard to which other systems can be compared.

2 1 0 3 2 0 3 0 3 2 4 0 4 1 0 2 0 0 1 0 2 0 1 0 0
2 2 0 4 2 4 0 2 2 1 0 0 0 1 0 2 0 0 0 2 1 0 0 0 0

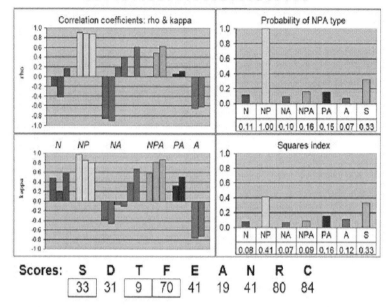

Scores:

S	D	T	F	E	A	N	R	C
33	31	9	70	41	19	41	80	84

The subject is female, age 51-60. Pregnancy, miscarriages.

Diagnosis: NP type

The test indicates a Dominant NP type with a low-moderate S score (33). As would be expected for a highly perfectionistic personality type, the focus F score of 70 is >> 50. The temperament T and extroversion E scores are low (9, 41), indicating a sociable, but reserved, individual.

The NPA model quite unexpectedly predicts *infertility* in parents of certain combinations of NPA types, namely in those couples who, because of their particular genotypes, are prone to conceive non-viable progeny totally lacking both traits N and A. We presume that a fetus lacking expression of both of these traits would not survive intrauterine life, appearing as a miscarriage or stillbirth, or would "fail to thrive" in early infancy [see Benis, 1985].

It can be shown that such infertility could occur only *in the mating of a non-aggressive type with a non-sanguine type*, namely N×A, N×PA, NP×A and NP×PA. Depending on the exact genotypes of the parents, infertility on the basis of such a "mismatch" could be partial or complete.

There are many possible reasons for miscarriages, but if our NP subject had a non-sanguine partner (A or PA type) then the reason for the infertility could be the genetic "mismatch" based on NPA personality type.

2 3 4 4 0 0 0 1 4 3 1 1 0 2 1 3 4 3 0 2 1 3 0 3 0
1 3 1 3 3 0 3 1 3 4 2 0 4 2 2 1 1 4 0 4 0 3 3 2 3

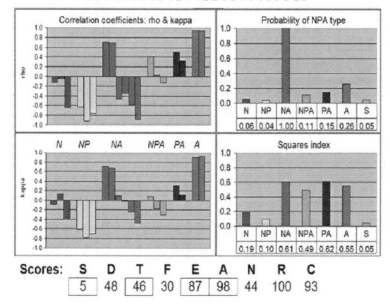

Scores:

S	D	T	F	E	A	N	R	C
5	48	46	30	87	98	44	100	93

Husband taking the test in place of his wife. Female, age 31-40. *This is in fact a test I did for my wife, a medium-size private enterprise owner in China, who admitted herself as "strong, harsh, picky, not tolerating others' flaws; self-centered, grandiose" ("People around me told me that I am [the above]")*

In a "surrogate test", one individual answers the questions of the test in place of another individual whom he or she knows very well.

Diagnosis: NA type

The test shows very low S score (5), low F score (30), and high T and E scores (46, 87), consistent with a Dominant NA type. The A score is also very high (98). The N score is relatively low (44), but this is because of a poor correlation of the subject's answers with those of a non-aggressive N type, not because of inhibition of trait N. The low F score (30) is concordant with the non-perfectionism of the NA type.

With the very high T, E and A scores, this is no doubt a very extroverted, aggressive individual, and there is very good agreement between the result of the test and the husband's description of his wife.

Note the similarity between this "surrogate test" and actual tests by individuals who gave test results of Dominant NA type (Cases 7, 8, 43, and 44).

2 0 0 3 0 1 0 1 2 1 0 4 3 1 0 3 3 3 1 1 3 0 0 2 0
0 3 0 0 0 1 0 4 3 4 3 1 0 3 2 0 3 1 3 4 2 0 2 3 1

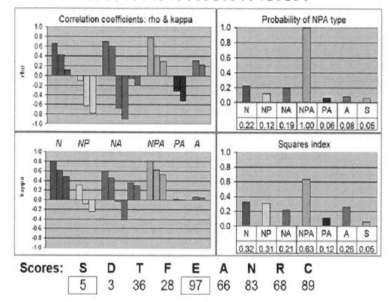

Scores:

S	D	T	F	E	A	N	R	C
5	3	36	28	97	66	83	68	89

(Russian version; Location: Turkey). Wife taking the test in place of her husband. Male, age 41-50. Depression, on medication. *Taken for husband* « для мужа ».

In a "surrogate test", one individual answers the questions of the test in place of another individual whom he or she knows very well.

Diagnosis: NPA+ type

The test shows very low S score (5), low F score (28), moderately high T score (36), and very high E score (97), consistent with a Dominant NPA+ type. The A score is moderately high (66). The N score is also elevated, reflective of fairly good correlation of the test with the Standard reference tests of the N group (especially N1).

The correlation coefficients were the highest for the NPA group (orange bars) for both the rho and kappa functions. With the near-maximum E score of 97, the test algorithm chose the NPA Dominant type.

It is interesting that this test comes from Turkey, which we had previously identified as a "Demonstrative habitancy" (a region having a high prevalence of NPA+ types). For further discussion of the geographic distribution of the NPA traits, see our monograph (Benis, 2017a).

For a comparison of this surrogate test with actual tests giving the NPA+ diagnosis, see Cases 9, 10 and 35.

1 1 2 1 0 0 3 1 0 1 2 1 4 0 1 3 1 0 3 2 1 0 2 1 0
0 0 0 4 0 3 0 0 0 0 2 0 2 1 0 4 0 0 1 3 1 0 0 1 0

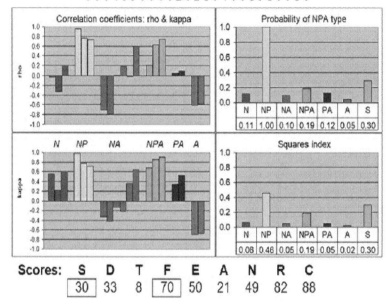

Scores:	S	D	T	F	E	A	N	R	C
	30	33	8	70	50	21	49	82	88

The subject is male, age 31-40. *I think the test is very accurate. However, I'd like to see more distinction between male and female behaviors in each personality type. As a child of a strong NA type, I have had many NA type women in my life, and they don't behave as NA-men would. Thank you for posting your test and research — they have changed my life! I have learned how to diagnose narcissists rapidly and accurately and can now install healthy personal boundaries and desires...*

Diagnosis: NP type

The test indicates a Dominant NP type with a low S score (30). As would be expected for a highly perfectionistic personality type, the focus F score of 70 is >> 50. The temperament T and extroversion E scores are low to moderate (8, 50), suggesting a sociable, but reserved, individual.

Of note is the subject's carefully-written comment with appropriate capitalization and punctuation, which would be typical of a perfectionistic NP type.

The subject's comment regarding "many NA women" in his is life is interesting, as NP types generally have an aversion to NA types (note the low Squares index for the NA category). Perhaps he meant women in a non-romantic context. Alternatively, one could consider the diagnosis of NPA−, but that seems unlikely in this case (see also Case 21).

40 NPA= type: masochist and slave

2 0 3 3 3 0 3 0 2 0 1 3 4 0 0 0 0 0 4 4 0 0 4 2 2
4 4 2 4 3 4 0 4 0 4 4 4 0 0 0 4 0 0 2 0 4 0 0 0 0

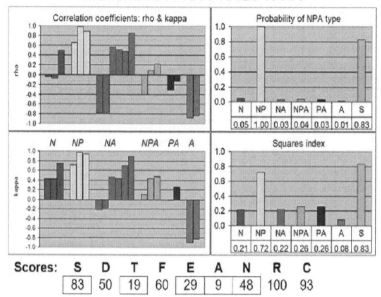

Scores:	S	D	T	F	E	A	N	R	C
	83	50	19	60	29	9	48	100	93

The subject is female, age 31-40. *Probably NP or NPA resigned or compliant. All 3 seem to fit. To a degree. Interestingly this is one of the first tests I've ever taken that mentions certain terms and proclivities. I am a physical masochist and I am a slave with a Master and a Husband. Many things I don't do well. Fitting in in the club environment, being a submissive, a slave, a wife, someone who balances the lives of 2 men, being a heavy bottom etc. These are all things I do well. Interesting...*

Diagnosis: NPA= type

The subject's test and comments are most consistent with the perfectionistic (compliant) Passive aggressive NPA= type, with a very high S score (83), and low T, E, A and N scores (19, 29, 9, 48). The F score of 60, being > 50 is consistent with the presence of the P trait. The low T, E, A and N scores, and the very high S score, suggest a very reserved individual, and in the context of self-reported masochism, socially a very submissive individual.

As we mentioned in Case 21 above, unbalanced relationships of dominance and submission based on the trait of aggression can readily occur with either partner being an A, NA, PA, NPA type, or even a Passive aggressive type. However, if a *Compliant* Passive aggressive type (NPA=, NA=, PA= or A=) is one of the partners, then he or she will always play the subservient role.

41 ADD with repressed aggression: English version

2 2 0 2 2 2 3 0 4 3 4 4 3 2 3 2 0 2 4 4 0 0 3 2 1
0 1 0 4 3 2 3 0 3 4 4 3 1 3 0 2 1 0 4 0 2 3 0 2 0

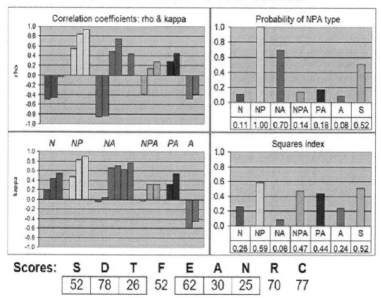

Scores:	S	D	T	F	E	A	N	R	C
	52	78	26	52	62	30	25	70	77

The subject is male, age 21-30. ADD, attention deficit disorder. *Diagnosed last year. I find your test very accurate, I define myself as a "repressed aggressive" person. I generally present a front of civism and citizenship, even kindness but I very often become angry for minor reason. I hold grudge and never forget even a minor slight. I sometime explode in fits of rage because of accumulated hostility.*

Diagnosis: NPA– type

The subject's test and comments are most consistent with the perfectionistic (non-compliant) Passive aggressive NPA– type with a moderately high S score (52), low-moderate T and E scores (26, 62), and low A and N scores (30, 25). The F score of 52 is consistent with the presence of the P trait. The low/moderate T, E, A and N scores, and the elevated S score, suggest a reserved individual.

Of note is the elevated detachment D score (78). Although the subject does not mention social withdrawal, the elevated D score is a hint that this individual is a former NPA– type who in the third decade of life is adopting "resignation" as a way of coping with the stresses of life. In that case, an alternative diagnosis would be "Resigned NP–A type". Finally, we note that with the moderate F score and the relatively high rho and kappa correlation coefficients in the NA group, the test algorithm did not eliminate NA– (or Resigned N–A) as a diagnostic possibility.

3 2 3 3 4 0 3 4 1 4 3 1 2 0 3 0 3 2 3 4 0 1 0 0 0
4 3 2 4 3 4 1 3 3 4 1 4 4 1 3 4 2 3 4 2 3 3 4 1 3

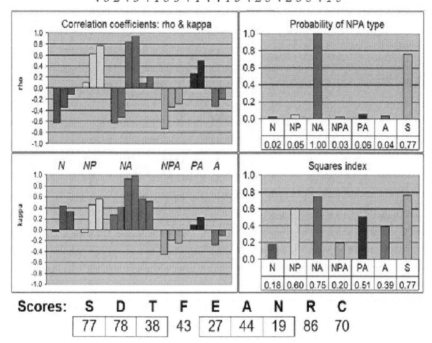

Scores:	S	D	T	F	E	A	N	R	C
	77	78	38	43	27	44	19	86	70

(Spanish version). The subject is female, age 21-30. ADD. *I was diagnosed as having passive aggressive personality.* ("Fui diagnosticada con personalidad pasiva agresiva")

Diagnosis: NA– type

The subject's test and comment regarding "passive aggressive personality" is most consistent with the non-perfectionistic (non-compliant) Passive aggressive NA– type with a high S score (77), low to moderate T and E scores (38, 27), and low A and N scores (44, 19). The low F score of 43 is consistent with the absence of the P trait. The low/moderate T, E, A and N scores, and the elevated S score, suggest a very reserved individual.

As in the preceding Case, of note is the elevated detachment D score (78). Although the subject does not comment on social withdrawal, the elevated D score is a hint that this individual is a former NA– type who in the third decade of life may be adopting "resignation" as a way of coping with the stresses of life. In that case, an alternative diagnosis would be "Resigned N–A type". Finally, we note that with the very high S score, this individual could be classified as a Compliant Passive aggressive NA= type with a tendency to social withdrawal.

Note that the NA– types differs from Compliant NA= types in that the latter always adopts the subservient role in social interactions.

4 4 2 4 0 4 0 0 0 4 4 4 0 0 4 4 4 4 2 0 0 4 0 4 0
0 4 0 0 4 0 1 2 4 4 1 0 4 0 0 0 3 4 0 4 0 4 1 0 4

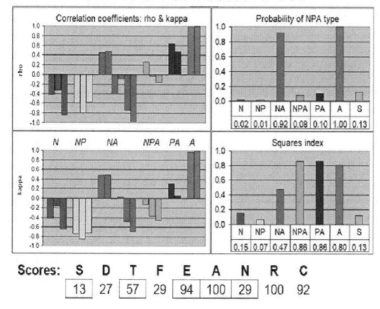

Scores:

S	D	T	F	E	A	N	R	C
13	27	57	29	94	100	29	100	92

The subject is male, age under 21. NPD (Narcissistic Personality Disorder). *I tend to lean towards antisocial also. Aggressive Narcissistism makes sense. I tend to be almost cut throat when there is something I want/need. I also also find myself scamming and manipulating situations to get around rules and through loopholes. Even before I knew about me having NPD I always admired some "interesting" characters, such as the high ups at Enron and other unsavory but rich and intelligent individuals.*

Diagnosis: A or NA type

The test shows very low S score (13), low F score (29), very high T and E scores (57, 94), and a maximum A score of 100 consistent with a Dominant A type. The N score is very low (29), which is to be expected for a non-sanguine A type (or for an aggressive NA type). The very low F score (29) is concordant with the non-perfectionism of the A type.

This individual is no doubt a very extroverted, aggressive individual who seems unembarrassed and unrepentant regarding his proclivities to antisocial behavior.

Of note is the fact that the test algorithm did not rule out the possibility of NA type (upper right graph). So, an alternative diagnosis would be "antisocial NA type". In fact, in our series of 100 internet test subjects giving the diagnosis of NPD, 76 gave test results of NA type.

4 1 3 4 0 4 3 4 4 1 0 4 0 0 4 4 4 4 1 4 0 1 1 1 0
4 4 3 0 4 0 4 3 4 4 4 3 4 2 0 1 1 0 1 3 4 4 1 0 0

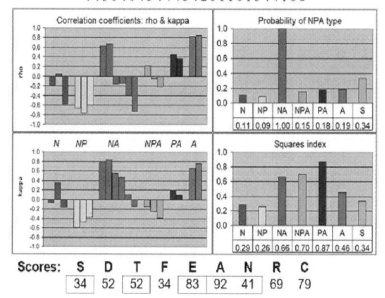

Scores:

S	D	T	F	E	A	N	R	C
34	52	52	34	83	92	41	69	79

The subject is male, age 51 to 60. NPD (Narcissistic Personality Disorder). *Some of the questions are problematic to respond to because they lump together many traits. EXAMPLES Question number 3 Is this you: talkative, impatient, much sex appeal, smiles and laughs easily, having a sharp-edged personality? Response – 3 I am talkative, impatient, ASEXUAL, smile and laugh but not that easily, and have a very sharp-edged (bordering on obnoxious) personality. Question number 7 Is this you: quiet, friendly...? Response – 3 I am NOISY, UNFRIENDLY, meticulous, extremely organized, aloof, nice smile, careful handwriting, WEAK and stubborn Otherwise, very interesting test! Sam*

Diagnosis: NA type

Shmuel "Sam" Vaknin, Israeli writer and author of "Malignant Self Love: Narcissism Revisited" (1999), kindly took the NPA test and allowed us to post the results. He provides us with the diagnosis of NPD.

Very similar to Case 43, the test shows low S score (34), high T and E scores (52, 83), and very high A score (92) consistent with a Dominant NA type. The N score is low (41), which reflects low correlation with the non-aggressive N category of the Standard reference tests. The low F score (34) is concordant with lack of P trait. Note that despite the similarity to Case 43, the test algorithm here eliminated "non-sanguine A type" as a possibility because of the greater response in the N and NA categories.

45 Asexual male: aloof NP type... or NP –A Resigned type?

3 1 0 1 3 0 2 0 3 3 3 4 4 2 3 3 0 2 4 4 0 0 2 2 2
0 2 0 4 3 2 3 0 0 4 4 3 0 3 0 3 2 0 4 0 2 3 0 3 1

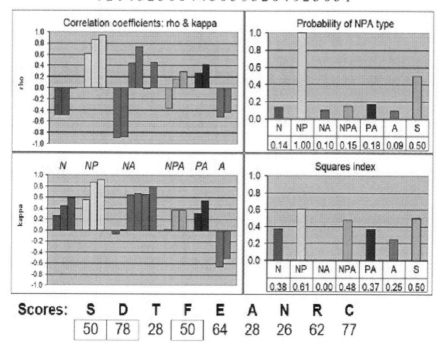

Scores:

S	D	T	F	E	A	N	R	C
50	78	28	50	64	28	26	62	77

The subject is male, age 21-30. *I am asexual (I do not see any interest in love relationships as well as casual sex, despite normal body features and hormone levels). Don't know if this can help you for further researches. Good luck anyway.*

Diagnosis: NP type (or NP –A Resigned type)

The test indicates a possible NP type with a moderate S score (50). The temperament T and extroversion E scores are moderate (28, 64), suggesting a somewhat reserved, individual. Note that the Squares index for the NA category is 0, meaning that this subject answered with "0" to all seven questions in the NA category. It is typical for placid NP types to have a disdain for the often frenetic temperament of NA types, and this is reflected in the aversion to answering positively to questions in the NA category. Of note is the subject's carefully-written comment, which would be typical of a perfectionistic NP type.

However, rather than an aloof NP type, two issues point to the alternative diagnosis of "NP –A Resigned type". First of all the focus F score of 50 would be borderline low for a highly perfectionistic NP personality type. Secondly, the detachment D score (78) is very high, suggesting that the subject is a former NPA– type who has incorporated "asexuality" into a life-style of resignation that he has not revealed to us.

2 2 0 0 0 0 2 0 2 2 0 3 1 0 3 1 1 0 1 1 2 0 0 0 0
0 2 2 3 2 0 0 1 0 0 0 0 1 0 0 0 0 0 1 0 0 2 0 0 0

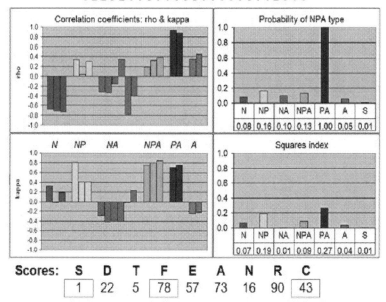

Scores:	S	D	T	F	E	A	N	R	C
	1	22	5	78	57	73	16	90	43

The subject is male, age under 21. Asthma. *I recently had a psychotic episode, and I am currently on antidepressants and antipsychotics (could have affected my results). I tried to be as consistent/honest as possible, and I have taken this test before.*

Diagnosis: PA type

The test shows Dominant (non-sanguine) PA type with very low S score (1). As would be expected for a highly perfectionistic personality type, the focus F score of 78 is >> 50. The moderately high A score (73) and the low N score (16) are consistent with a Dominant non-sanguine PA type. The temperament T and extroversion E scores are low (5, 57), indicating a Dominant, but reserved, individual.

Of note is the low C score of statistical consistency (43), and the high value of kappa in the NP group (0.80), suggesting that the alternative diagnosis of Dominant (sanguine) NP type should also be considered.

The subject does not mention any family history of mental illness, but such is common for PA types with psychotic disorders (see Case 12 above). In accordance with NPA genetics: 1) non-sanguine types tend to cluster in families, and 2) NPA types having only one of the traits, N or A, are more prone to psychosis in comparison to Dominant NA or NPA+ types. For a further discussion of how the NPA traits are transmitted and how they impinge on the heritability of schizophrenia, see the Bibliography.

1 0 4 3 4 0 3 0 0 0 2 2 3 3 2 3 3 0 4 4 4 0 4 2 2
2 0 0 2 2 4 1 4 4 2 3 4 0 3 0 1 0 0 0 2 3 3 2 3 0

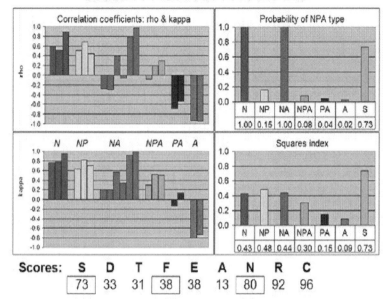

Scores:

S	D	T	F	E	A	N	R	C
73	33	31	38	38	13	80	92	96

(French version). The subject is female, age less than 21. Panic disorder. *Hypersensitive, eczema, panic attacks, shy at first but outgoing immediately after (once being at ease with to the other person) active, need my own world to me but need others, afraid of feeling scared and afraid of being alone.*

« Hypersensible, eczema, panique, timide au premier abord expansive tout de suite après (une fois à l'aise selon l'autre personne) active, besoin de mon monde à moi mais besoin des autres, peur du sentiment peur et peur d'être seule »

Diagnosis: NA= type

The test indicates (compliant) Passive aggressive NA= type with a very high S score (73), moderate T score (31), low E score (38), very low A score (13), and low F score (38). The N score is elevated (80).

In general, the NA= type is differentiated from the NA− type mainly by the higher S score (> 70) in the NA= type. Given the high N score, this test might also be consistent with an "N type with high S score", which in our notation would be N– or –N, i.e. a Borderline N type.

The subject reports eczema, which we have previously linked to high S score, or A–/= trait. Interestingly, there is research literature on a relation between eczema (atopic dermatitis) and panic disorder.

0 0 0 1 3 0 1 0 1 0 1 1 2 4 0 0 1 0 4 4 1 1 4 0 0
0 0 1 1 0 4 1 1 1 1 2 4 0 0 2 4 0 0 1 3 4 1 0 0 0

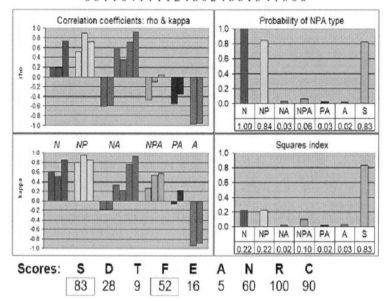

Scores:

S	D	T	F	E	A	N	R	C
83	28	9	52	16	5	60	100	90

The subject is female, age under 21. *i cry at night only, before i go to sleep, and i don't know why*

Diagnosis: Borderline N− type (or NA= Compliant type)

The test shows "N or NP type" with very high S score (83), moderate F score (52) and very low T, E and A scores (9, 16, 5). In the context of a young individual, this would be the Borderline N− or N− P type.

The N− and N− P types are typically non-aggressive, docile individuals differentiated primarily by the presence or absence of perfectionistic behavior. We do not have any hard information regarding this subject's behavior, but the non-perfectionistic nature of her comment would point to the non-perfectionistic N− type rather than N− P type.

Furthermore, in the test results above: 1) the F score of 52 would be near the lower limit of what one would expect for an NP type, and 2) the rho and kappa correlation coefficient values in the N and NA/NA− groups are in the same neighborhood as the values for the NP group. Hence, the test algorithm understandably favored N– type over N– P type.

Previously in Borderline types (Chap. 7), we saw cases where the detachment D score was high, suggesting aloofness. However, that is not the case here: despite the high S score and low T, E and A scores indicating docility, there is no evidence of a tendency to social withdrawal.

4 0 4 4 0 4 0 0 3 3 1 3 0 0 3 4 4 4 2 3 1 0 0 3 3
4 0 0 4 3 1 2 1 0 3 3 0 0 3 0 1 0 3 2 3 3 4 4 4 1

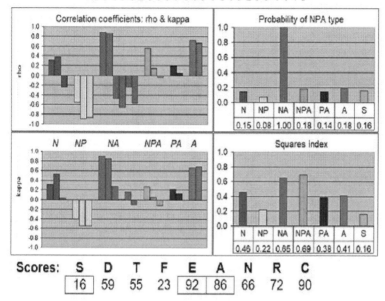

Scores: S   D   T   F   E   A   N   R   C
         16   59   55   23   92   86   66   72   90

The subject is male, age 41 to 50. ADHD. *I test in the NA, but according to synopsis, I am closer to NPA. I was a good provider for many years, worked independently with clients for many years and my dressing style fits with NPA rather than NA.*

Diagnosis: NPA+ type with ADHD

The tests shows apparent NA type with low S score (16), high T score (55), low F score (23), very high E score (92) and high A score (86).

The subject believes that he is an NPA+ type, with the test giving a mistaken diagnosis of NA type. We believe that, indeed, he may be correct. Although the test algorithm eliminated NPA+ type as the diagnosis, the highest Squares index was of the NPA+ category and the rho correlation coefficient for NPA+ was a respectable 0.55.

The subject's succinct comment that he takes pride in having been a reliable family man is concordant with what one would expect from an earnest NPA+ type, and it does not have the chatty style often seen in the comments by N or NA types. The remark regarding dressing style is also telling: NPA+ types look in disdain at the more ostentatious, colorful wardrobes of their NA cousins.

We conclude that an NPA+ type who is (by other genes) predisposed to ADHD can have the superficial behavior and Test results of "NA type".

CHAPTER 9

Summary

- The NPA model is based on the three genetic traits of sanguinity (N), perfectionism (P) and aggression (A).

- The model generates discrete personality types in the categories of Dominant, Passive aggressive, Resigned/ Detached, and Borderline.

- The NPA personality test consists of 50 questions, each of which requires a numerical answer from 0 to 4.

- The 50 questions are partitioned into 7 categories: the six Dominant types (N, NP, NA, NPA, PA, A) and a seventh category (S) characterizing non-dominance, or inhibition of the traits N and/or A.

- Seven *Squares indexes,* normalized to a maximum value of unity, are computed. They represent the intensity of the subject's response in each of the 7 test categories.

- Nine *Test scores* are computed, each scaled to a maximum value of 100. These are: S (non-dominance, or submissiveness), D (resignation, or detachment), T (temperament), F (focus), E (extroversion), A (aggression), N (sanguinity, or narcissism), R (coherence, or consistency of response to the questions) and C (statistical consistency).

- The test algorithm is a computational scheme based on Boolean logic that decides on the most probable NPA diagnosis, which is defined to have a probability of 1. The algorithm demotes an NPA diagnostic category if any one of the quantitative criteria for that category is violated.

- The algorithm decides on the most probable NPA diagnosis by comparing the subject's answers to 19 composite Standard reference tests with the use of 1) correlation coefficients and other statistical functions, and 2) the seven Squares indexes and the nine Test scores.

- In Chaps. 4 to 8, forty-nine representative test results are presented in the categories of Dominant, Passive aggressive, Resigned/ Detached and Borderline types. These are actual tests taken online that were submitted to us, and many of them are accompanied by the subject's comments.

- The test results are presented in a standard abridged form, consisting of graphical displays of 1) the NPA diagnosis by the computer algorithm, 2) the Squares indexes for the seven categories of questions, and 3) two sets of the correlation coefficients, rho and kappa, that compare the subject's response to the 19 Standard reference tests.

- The reader is invited to take the NPA test online at npatheory.com, with comments being welcome.

APPENDIX A
Details of the NPA test

Fig. A1. The NPA test as it appears on the web page. Each of the 50 questions requires an answer from 0 to 4 on the dropdown list. →

NPA PERSONALITY TEST

This is a 50-question test to assist in the determination of your NPA Character Type.
The charts below will display when all questions are answered. Instant results!

All questions are answered on a 0 to 4 scale, as follows:

4 = "I agree" or TRUE or Yes!
3 = "I somewhat agree"
2 = Neutral
1 = "I somewhat disagree"
0 = "I disagree" or FALSE or No!

Suggestions: Take a bit of time before answering. Imagine the situations depicted.
Think about yourself rather than about the test. Try to see yourself as others see you. Read the entire list of questions before starting the test.

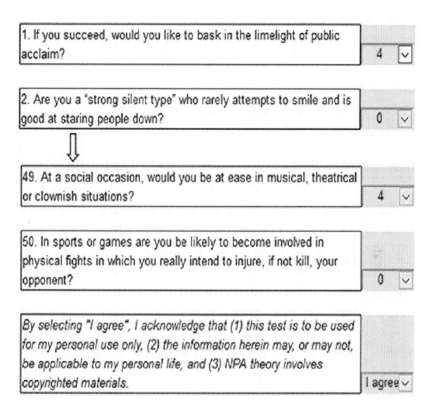

APPENDIX A

Details of the NPA test

The 50 questions

The test, as it is displayed on the web page, is shown in Fig, A1, above. For the test questions in five other languages, see *Appendix B.*

The fifty questions of the test are listed below:

1. If you succeed, would you like to bask in the limelight of public acclaim?

2. Are you a "strong silent type" who rarely attempts to smile and is good at staring people down?

3. Is this you: talkative, impatient, much sex appeal, smiles and laughs easily, having a sharp-edged personality?

4. When things must get done, are you liable to push people aside and

ask questions later?

5. With minor stress, do you have a tremulous voice or hesitancy in speech?

6. At a quiet party, would you welcome a newcomer with a hearty yell across the room?

7. Is this you: quiet, friendly, meticulous, extremely organized, aloof, nice smile, careful handwriting, strong and stubborn?

8. Does your laughter tend to the high-pitched, hysterical side?

9. Do you tend to be suspicious and confrontational, rather than accepting other people's motives and actions?

10. In a touching, emotional situation, would you be unsympathetic to the "weeping weaklings" around you and head for the door?

11. In school were you an earnest, introspective student who was hesitant to speak up in class, dying a thousand deaths waiting to be called upon?

12. In relaxed social situations, do you speak with a loud, carefully-controlled voice and make intense eye contact with others?

13. Are you attracted to activities that are slow moving and require careful attention to detail?

14. In school or college would you be attracted to cheerleading, singing, drama or the dance?

15. On the stage would you be natural as the villain: cool, calculating, suspicious, vindictive, a stern colorless face, and a dagger at hand?

16. Do you have the potential to be a well-organized, dynamic speaker who would never read to an audience from a prepared text?

17. Could you be described as hyperactive, unembarrassable, and attracted to good food, sex, travel and excitement?

18. Is it possible that you will tangle with the law for vindictive, belligerent, violent behavior?

19. When "wronged" by someone, do you typically reply with "the silent treatment" rather than being vocal?

20. Do you sometimes "get into a world of your own", become

depressed and think that you could survive as a hermit?

21. In photographs do you and at least one family member show a broad charismatic smile?

22. Could this be you: loud, unrestrained, unsmiling, colorless complexion, tendency to bully, unfocused, unruly, a real brute?

23. Are you a nice person who is easily taken advantage of, or bullied, in work or love relationships?

24. Is this you: sociable but not sexy, rather loud voice, conventional lifestyle, maternalistic or paternalistic, dynamic, a managerial outlook on life, a bulldog?

25. Do these terms apply to you: extroverted, unaggressive, unfocused, warm, vain, sexy, unconventional: a teddy bear or a baby doll?

26. When excited does your voice easily become piercing (male) or shrill (female)?

27. When you have a seething rage, does the blood drain from your face, giving you a frightening, evil appearance?

28. Do people say, much to your annoyance, that you have the "clean gene", or that you are "obsessive-compulsive"?

29. Are you rather slow to be drawn into intimate or sexual relationships?

30. Could this be you: reserved, well organized, aloof, tending to be sarcastic or cynical, a grin rather than a smile, a coiled spring capable of pouncing on someone?

31. Do you get extremely nervous or anxious about speaking in public, even in benign situations?

32. Are you an extroverted, active person who has no interest at all in social events or friendly people?

33. Do you become more upset than most people if there is a lack of order, neatness or cleanliness?

34. When angered, could you be described as tearful, hysterical, and liable to lash out with talons bared?

35. If someone were slow at doing something, would you immediately intervene and say with a forceful voice, "Let me help you with that!"

36. At a party can you become really carried away while telling people about your interests and expertise?

37. Do you generally lack self-confidence or have feelings of free-floating anxiety or inferiority?

38. Would you do well in the imagined role of a stern, pallid-faced Roman emperor (empress) capable of harsh judgments?

39. Could you picture yourself as the TV anchorperson: likeable, reserved smile, very organized, very focused, forceful voice: a really dynamic individual?

40. Does colorful adornment, e.g., fancy clothes, rings or accessories of gold, come naturally to you?

41. Are you shy in social situations, e.g., small groups, parties, dinners?

42. If someone were casually to lay a hand on you, is it likely that you would immediately respond with a punch in the face?

43. Are you rather likely to have many short-lived love affairs in which you treat your weaker partner rather cruelly?

44. Are you rather slow and very stubborn in getting a task well done?

45. Are you (potentially) a good leader because of your dynamic style, your talents for organization, as well as your ease in social situations?

46. Do you go at lengths to avoid anxiety-producing confrontations with other people?

47. Is your humor reserved, biting and sarcastic, rather than open and jocular?

48. Are you more hyperactive and sexually provocative than other people, a vampire in your dreams?

49. At a social occasion, would you be at ease in musical, theatrical or clownish situations?

50. In sports or games are you likely to become involved in physical fights in which you really intend to injure, if not kill, your opponent?

Demographic information

Test subjects are given the option to identify their gender and age, and also to specify from a dropdown list any medical or other condition that they might have. There is also a text box where comments may be entered.

Categorization of the questions

The 50 questions are divided into six categories of Dominant types (7 questions each) and a seventh group defining the S category of non-dominance (8 questions), as follows:

Dominant types

    N type: # 1, 14, 21, 25, 36, 40, 49

    NP type: # 7, 13, 19, 28, 29, 33, 44

    NA type: # 3, 8, 17, 26, 34, 43, 48

    NPA type: # 6, 12, 16, 24, 35, 39, 45

    PA type: # 2, 9, 15, 27, 30, 38, 47

    A type: # 4, 10, 18, 22, 32, 42, 50

Non-dominance

    S category: # 5, 11, 20, 23, 31, 37, 41, 46

Squares indexes

Squares indexes are calculated as the sum of the squares of the response values in each of the above categories, each normalized to the maximum value of unity. A Squares index of unity for a category indicates that the subject answered the highest value of "4" for all the seven or eight questions of that category.

Test scores

The S, D, T, F and E test scores are computed arithmetically from the sums of squares of the answers in the relevant categories. The A, N, R and C scores are computed from coefficients of correlation between answers of the test subject and those of the Standard tests. All test scores are scaled, or normalized, to range from 0 to 100.

S score

The score is derived from the sums of squares (*ss*) of the answers to the eight questions of the S category.

The S score is presumed to be a non-specific measure of *non-dominance*, or lack of genetic full expression of the N or A traits. It is can also reflect *anxiety, depression* or *submissiveness* in social relations due to environmental stress. If the S score is greater than 20-30 then it becomes more likely that the traits N and/or A are not fully expressed, either because of genetics or environment.

S score < 20 — the test is presumed to be consistent with a Dominant type (N, A, NA, NP, PA or A).

..... *20 to 30* — transition region

..... *30 to 75* — the presumed diagnosis is non-compliant Passive aggressive type (NA–, NPA–, PA–, and A–) or Non-aggressive Borderline type (such as N– or N–P).

..... *> 75* — the presumed diagnosis is compliant Passive aggressive type (such as NA= or NPA=) or Non-aggressive Borderline type (such as N– or N– P / N= or N=P).

D score

The score is derived from the *ss* of questions # 10, 20, 29, 32.

The D score is a measure of *detachment* or social avoidance. It is used to establish the diagnosis of Resigned type and may be elevated in Borderline types.

The correspondence of typical values is as follows:

D score 0 to 50 — low tendency to detachment.

..... *50 to 75* — moderate tendency to detachment.

..... *> 75* — high tendency to detachment, as in the Resigned types (such as N –A, NP –A).

The categories of Dominant types, together with the S and D scores that identify non-dominant types, are the basis of our analysis of the "idealized" response to the test as detailed in Chapter 2.

T score

The score is derived from the *ss* of the answers to questions of the four N, NA, NPA and A Dominant categories. Thus, the T score uses 28 questions of the test.

The T score is presumed to be a measure of *temperament*. Reserved individuals will tend to score low on this scale, while highly extroverted, volatile subjects will tend to score high. Presence of the P trait tends to reduce the T score. Low T scores are seen in the Passive aggressive and Borderline types. The highest scores are seen in Dominant NA types. The types having the widest variability of T scores are also the NA types.

The correspondence of typical values is as follows:

T score 0 to 10 — low, reticent
..... 10 to 20 — low, reserved
..... 20 to 35 — moderate temperament
..... 35 to 60 — high, reactive
..... 60 to 100 — high, volatile

F score

The F score is calculated from the ratio of the *ss* of the answers to questions of the perfectionistic NP and PA categories to the total *ss* of all six Dominant categories. Thus, the F score uses 42 questions of the test.

The F score, for *focus*, is presumed to be a measure of the degree of organization of an individual's personality. Introverted, reserved and perfectionistic individuals with analytical tendencies will tend to score high on this scale, while less focused, expansive or practical individuals will tend to score low. Types lacking the P trait are unlikely to score higher than an F score of 55. The highest scores are seen in the NP and PA Dominant types, and in the perfectionistic Inhibited aggressive and Borderline types.

The correspondence of typical values is as follows:

F score 0 to 20 — low, diffuse, expansive
..... 20 to 70 — moderate, reflective, pragmatic
..... 70 to 100 — high, contemplative, analytical

E score

The E score for "extroversion" is calculated from the subject's positive *ss* response in the NPA+ category (seven questions) and lack of *ss* response in the S category of non-dominance (eight questions). The score gives equal weight to the *ss* of the seven responses in the NPA+ category and the *ss* of the eight responses of in the S category. The E score is scaled so that an NPA Dominant type will have an E score close to 100, while a Compliant Passive aggressive type or Borderline type will score close to 0.

The correspondence of typical values is as follows:

E score 0 to 30 — low, introverted

..... 30 to 70 — moderate

..... 70 to 100 — high, extroverted

A score

The A score for "aggression" is proportional to the rho/kappa values corresponding to the correlation of the test answers with those of the Standard test of the Dominant A type (Standard tests A1, A2). The score is normalized to a scale of 0 to 100, corresponding to rho/kappa values of −1 and +1, respectively. Values of A score less than 50 indicate either lack or inhibition of trait A, or presence of the modulating trait P.

The correspondence of typical values is as follows:

A score 0 to 30 — very low aggression

..... 30 to 50 — low, suppressed aggression

..... 50 to 70 — moderate to high aggression

..... 70 to 100 — high assertiveness or overt aggression in A or NA type

N score

The N score for sanguinity or "narcissism" is proportional to the rho value corresponding to the correlation of the test answers with those of the Standard test of the Dominant N type (Standard test N1). The score is normalized to a scale of 0 to 100, corresponding to rho values of −1 and +1, respectively. Values of N score less than 50 indicate either lack or inhibition of trait N, or presence of the modulating trait P.

The correspondence of typical values is as follows:

N score 0 to 30 — absent N trait
..... 30 to 40 — transition zone
..... 40 to 60 — variable narcissistic behavior
..... 60 to 85 — high probability of N trait
..... 85 to 100 — high sociability or overt narcissism in N or NA type

R score

The R score for "consistency of response to questions," or "coherence", is computed from the maximum value plus the standard deviation of the 19 values of the r function. Thus, if a subject gives test answers (0 to 4) in a completely random fashion, then there should be no correlation between the subject's answers and any of the Standard tests. The 19 values of the correlation coefficient r should cluster around a mean of 0 with a very small standard deviation. The possible range of the R score is scaled from 0 to 100. See also Case 33 in Chap. 8.

A low value of R score could have many possible explanations, such as inattentiveness, immaturity, intelligence, language difficulties, trying to "beat the test", not responding truthfully to sensitive questions, trying to give a pleasing or exceptional result, deciding to answer the questions with a particular strategy, and many other reasons as well.

The correspondence of typical values is as follows:

R score 0 to 50 — random or exceptional response
..... 50 to 65 — transition zone
..... 65 to 100 — consistent response

C score

The C score for "statistical consistency", is computed from the correlation coefficient between the 19 pairs of values of the rho and kappa functions. Since the rho and kappa functions depend on the r and J functions, respectively, the C score is taken as a measure of how well the four statistical computations agree with each other.

In general, if the R score of a test is low, the statistical consistency reflected in the C score will be low, as well. The C score is scaled from 0 to 100. A value of the C score of 0 would correspond to a zero or negative correlation coefficient between the rho and kappa functions, i.e., no agreement between the results of the two statistical functions.

The correspondence of typical values is as follows:

C score 0 to 60 — low statistical consistency

..... 60 to 75 — moderate consistency

..... 75 to 100 — good statistical consistency

Use of the rho and kappa functions

The NPA test uses correlation coefficients in several ways. In particular, the *r function* generates sets of nineteen *50-point* correlation coefficients that directly compare the subject test answers to those of the 19 Standard tests, while the *rho* and *kappa functions* generate sets of *19-point* correlation coefficients that compare the subject's r and J profiles to those of the 19 Standard tests. Thus, the rho and kappa functions measure the agreement between paired values in 19 categories. In so doing, the rho and kappa functions usually act as more sensitive measures of agreement between the subject's answers and the Standard tests than does the r function. To illustrate this with the use of Test Example 5 of Chap. 3, the figure below compares the values of the r and rho functions for the 19 categories of the Standard tests. It can be seen that the r function values, whether positive or negative, are amplified in the rho function.

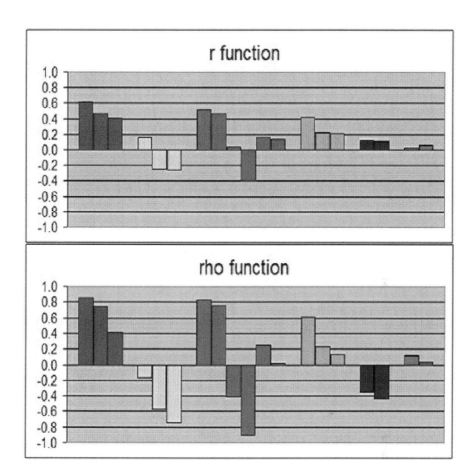

Use of r-squared, rho-squared and kappa-squared values

In classical statistics, *r-squared* is a statistical measure of how close the data cluster to the fitted regression line. Intuitively, we interpret *r-squared*, *rho-squared* and *kappa-squared* values in the sense of "probability of concordance between the subject's test answers and those of the Standard tests". Hence, we use the term "probability of NPA type" in this limited sense only.

Printed in Great Britain
by Amazon

28449570R00094